S0-EAY-466

THE HEALTH
OF AMERICANS

C.P. Thomson

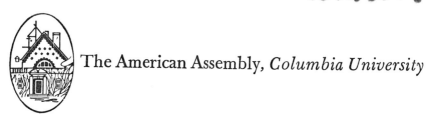

The American Assembly, *Columbia University*

THE HEALTH
OF AMERICANS

Prentice-Hall, Inc., *Englewood Cliffs, N. J.*

A SPECTRUM BOOK

Copyright © 1970 by The American Assembly, Columbia University, under International and Pan-American Copyright Conventions. All rights reserved. No part of this book may be reproduced in any form or by any means without permission in writing from the publisher. C–13-385070-6; P–13-385062-5. *Library of Congress Catalog Card Number 70-120793.*

Printed in the United States of America.

Current printing (last number):

10 9 8 7 6 5 4 3 2 1

PRENTICE-HALL INTERNATIONAL, INC. (*London*)
PRENTICE-HALL OF AUSTRALIA, PTY. LTD. (*Sydney*)
PRENTICE-HALL OF CANADA, LTD. (*Toronto*)
PRENTICE-HALL OF INDIA PRIVATE LIMITED (*New Delhi*)
PRENTICE-HALL OF JAPAN, INC. (*Tokyo*)

Preface

Boisfeuillet Jones, president of the Emily and Ernest Woodruff Foundation, Atlanta, Georgia, on consultation with a number of authorities in the field of health, laid out the program for the Thirty-seventh American Assembly. He outlined the critical issues and on behalf of the Assembly engaged the writers of the chapters which follow—chapters offered as background reading for the participants in the Arden House Assembly, April 23–26, 1970, on *The Health of Americans*. The Assembly, a heterogeneous group of some seventy laymen and health professionals, thought and talked about the subject for three days and then declared their views in a summary report. Published as a pamphlet, the report has been circulated in large numbers across the nation and may be had from The American Assembly.

The volume at hand is meant for the general public, and for use as background reading for all regional American Assemblies held across the nation under the sponsorship of other educational institutions.

The Richard King Mellon Charitable Trusts, The Commonwealth Fund, The Rockefeller Foundation, The Laurel Foundation, and the Leon Falk Family Trust all contributed to financial support of this program (the proportion related to order of listing), for which The American Assembly is deeply grateful. The donors, however, have no stake in the outcome of this project; and neither has The American Assembly, a national nonpartisan educational organization. The views herein belong to the authors themselves.

Clifford C. Nelson
President
The American Assembly

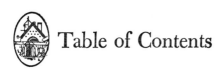 Table of Contents

Boisfeuillet Jones, Editor
Introduction   1

1   *Julius B. Richmond*
Human Development   5

2   *William H. Stewart*
Health Assessment   39

3   *Howard P. Rome*
Mental Health   65

4   *William N. Hubbard, Jr.*
Health Knowledge   93

5   *James L. Goddard*
Health Protection   121

6   *James Z. Appel*
Health Care Delivery   141

7   *Herman M. Somers*
Health Care Cost   167

Index   205

The American Assembly   211

THE HEALTH
OF AMERICANS

Boisfeuillet Jones, Editor

Introduction

The health of Americans is better than ever before, as we enter the last three decades of the twentieth century. But our health could and should be much better—we demand it and expect it. Why do we not have it? Seven authorities explain why in this book.

A definition of health as the complete physical, mental, and social well-being of an individual is generally accepted. Dr. Richmond explains the meaning of this definition in terms of full human development. Modern medicine has concentrated appropriately on the study and control of disease, but attention must now be given to the positive concept of health maintenance as the manifestation of optimal human development. He suggests that human developmental processes may have more significance for health in the future than disease. His essential theme is that optimal human development is a result of the interaction of genetic potentialities with a favorable environment.

BOISFEUILLET JONES *was the nation's chief health official in 1961–64 as special assistant to the secretary (health and medical affairs), Department of Health, Education and Welfare. In 1965 he was executive vice chairman of The White House Conference on Health, and in 1967–68 chairman of the President's Advisory Commission on Health Facilities. Former vice president and administrator of health services at Emory University, Mr. Jones has been consultant or member of a number of other advisory groups in the field of health, including the Advisory Group to the Surgeon General on Environmental Health (chairman), the delegation to study medicine in the Soviet Union (chairman), the Committee of Consultants on Medical Research for the U.S. Senate (chairman), and the National Advisory Health Council. He is now president of the Emily and Ernest Woodruff Foundation, Atlanta.*

The accepted definition of health is an abstraction and cannot be measured in objective terms. Dr. Stewart discusses this in describing the burden of disease, injury, and ill-health as reflected in objective statistics. He indicates that changes in these statistics for the better will be modest and that further change will occur when knowledge is developed permitting the large-scale prevention of such major conditions as heart disease or prematurity and immaturity at birth. New methods need to be constructed toward better measurement of health beyond the specific current use of national morbidity and mortality data.

Mental illness traditionally has been avoided as a condition to be dealt with medically. Although separation of physical and mental health is not justified in considering the health of an individual, the heavy incidence of mental problems and the new techniques for dealing with them justify special discussion of the subject. Dr. Rome traces the history of mental illness from avoidance to meaningful medical involvement. He emphasizes that mental health involves not only professional psychiatrists and psychologists, but the whole social fabric. He makes it clear that for the most part mental and emotional illness represents patterns of reaction in a given social and cultural environment to the myriad of factors which influence an individual. Identifying and dealing with these factors is essential for prevention as well as treatment.

Many of us have almost unlimited expectations of health improvement through application of vast new knowledge and techniques for prevention and treatment of disease. Dr. Hubbard explains the limitations of such knowledge, the procedures required for continuing the outpouring of knowledge from effective research, and the limitations of health manpower, training, and utilization. He describes the biomedical research effort and reports a frame of reference for health knowledge; he describes particular health problems illustrating that fundamental and applied biological knowledge have great usefulness in improving man's health. The application of knowledge finds expression through the manpower available to deliver such knowledge. He explains the process for training professional health manpower, with relation to shortages.

Hazards to health from products in the market and from the environment have become serious national concerns only recently. Dr. Goddard deals with the full spectrum of such hazards and describes the resources for and the nature of protection against them. He raises several basic questions concerning planning and responsibility in the areas of research and protection, using the detonation of the first hydrogen bomb as an example of massive, traumatic assault by man upon the environment—and upon his fellow man. Doctor Goddard describes the three environments—personal, immediate, and general—in which the individual may be under attack. He suggests certain major concerns for study and relates them to an awareness among youth that environmental health protection is a priority for the next generation of public leadership.

Demands for health care exceed the supply of services for many people in many areas. Dr. Appel recognizes limitations of the current health care delivery arrangements and suggests modifications which offer hope of more effective and efficient health care without destroying the strengths on which present activities are based. His principal theme concerns the lack of community systems for continuity of care—the need for providing a full spectrum of services available to all individuals and their families where they live. The specialization of health professionals and the independent management of related health facilities have tended to inhibit attention to the whole person in maintenance of health and prevention of disease. He suggests ways in which the system of delivering services may better recognize the needs of individuals for comprehensive care, rather than emphasizing treatment of disease categories or separate parts of the body and utilizing inappropriate facilities for the type of care indicated.

Costs of health care have accelerated dramatically in recent years. Professor Somers analyzes the reasons and suggests possibilities for cost controls. With a practical limitation on the public and private dollars which can be committed to health purposes, improvement of health has direct relation to the value received for each dollar invested. He points out that effective analysis and control of costs must take account of the need for better means of financing health care, more effective and efficient delivery of services, and equitable availability of care, as well as the external economy. We also face such issues as deciding how limitations will be placed on enormously expensive procedures from developing technologies which have effective life-saving potential.

Simply, the book suggests seven elements for health improvement:

1. An understanding of human development in relation to daily living.
2. Better methodology with which to assess the nation's health and guide its efforts.
3. Acceptance of emerging knowledge about mental conditions and behavioral patterns as guides to individual care and social action.
4. Strengthening of efforts toward production of health knowledge and utilization of such knowledge through education of health personnel.
5. Recognition and control of environmental hazards to health.

6. Organization of health services into community systems for comprehensive care available to all.

7. Better and fairer means of financing and more efficient delivery of health care, and relation of health care costs to investments in the quality of the living environment.

The reader will recognize recurring basic themes in this presentation: health maintenance through education and prevention requires emphasis; low income has a direct relation to poor health; maldistributed and fractionated health services need correction through efficient organization; health involves interaction between biological and environmental factors, with increasing emphasis on the environment; enormous health benefits lie ahead from further research; new health knowledge and technology will require new dimensions of judgment from society as to who receives benefits; and others.

The book suggests to readers, lay and professional, what we as a people can do and ought to do to improve our health—and how to do it. Further, it implies a deterioration in health unless we move constructively now.

Julius B. Richmond

1

Human Development

An implicit goal of our society is the enhancement of each person's opportunity for a healthy, reasonably happy, and productive life. The pursuit of this goal depends upon our knowledge of human development and the provision of an environment and services which foster optimal development. For our purposes, human development includes the cultural, social, and psychological as well as biological aspects of growth and development. And since, in the eyes of professional observers of growth and development, these processes are so related, the terms *growth* and *development* are used interchangeably.

That we do not fully respect the value we implicitly place on human life is apparent in our recent history: although knowledge of human development has increased, application of that knowledge has not kept pace. Thus, with the sociological changes emphasized by urbanization and technological advances, there has been a substantial deterioration in man's environment. Air and water pollution, radiation hazards, crowding, poor housing, inadequate transportation systems and consequent high accident rates, and inappropriate use of pesticides, detergents, and drugs are but a few of the problems which impede man's

JULIUS B. RICHMOND, M.D., *is dean of the Medical Faculty and chairman of the Department of Pediatrics, State University of New York, Upstate Medical Center, Syracuse. Dr. Richmond has won several distinguished service awards for his many written works and lectures and numerous acts of public and private service in human development. He was chairman of the Committee on Adolescence for the World Health Organization, and in 1965–1966 was national director of Project Head Start and the Office of Health Affairs of the Office of Economic Opportunity.*

5

fulfillment of his greatest potentialities. It is apparent that concern over human development is not the province of the health professions and agencies exclusively; rather all those concerned with education, welfare, transportation, housing, agriculture and food processing, and many others have significant responsibilities bearing on health and human development. Health is a major concern, since it is the manifestation of optimal human development.

The Concept of Health and Human Development

The health professions until recently have given little attention to health as a positive concept. This is understandable, since it is little more than one hundred years ago that modern medicine had its origins around the study of disease under the influence of the pathologist Virchow. This was made possible by the development of the microscope. Cellular pathology became a dominant theme in medicine, and by the turn of the century advances in the natural sciences led to the addition of biochemistry, physiology, microbiology, and pharmacology to medical education and to the establishment of the modern medical school curriculum.

The focus on disease has led to the brilliant advances in modern medical knowledge which have provided us with a better understanding and control over the infectious, metabolic, and nutritional disorders so prevalent in the early years of this century. New treatment approaches, including advances in surgery and such procedures as renal dialysis, are succeeding in prolonging life. While these advances create new complexities in medicine and require large professional staffs, the demands have been balanced in part by the conservation of professional manpower through the preventive practices which have evolved. We need only think of the large numbers of health professionals who were busy caring for children with rickets, scurvy, whooping cough, diphtheria, tetanus, measles, and poliomyelitis—diseases which have largely been eliminated in the United States—to become aware of some of the manpower savings which have been accomplished.

It would seem appropriate, therefore, that segments of the health professions attend more directly to the problems of conserving or maintaining health—or fostering optimal human development. The World Health Organization recognized this need when it defined health as "a state of physical and mental well-being and not merely the absence of disease."

But the health professions, heavily rooted in the study of disease,

are not conceptually well-equipped to study health. Although our vocabulary and classification of disease are well developed, we have
virtually no vocabulary or classification of functional capacity in
health. Particularly in relationship to social and psychological effectiveness, we have only the crudest kind of language and no classification of man's capacity to cope with his environment. Dr. Karl Menninger has given some recognition to this problem by utilizing such
terms as "wellness" to contrast with sickness, and "weller-than-well"
to describe a higher order of effectiveness.

It may be that the health professions of the future will be oriented
more toward developmental processes than diseases. Indeed, this is
already taking place as the new knowledge of genetics, biochemistry,
immunology, and microbiology provides more techniques by which
we can understand each human being more fully, anticipate the developmental hazards to which he may be predisposed, and hopefully
intercept these hazards. In the process, medicine will need to shift some
of its institutional base from the hospital to the community in order
to observe people who are considered healthy. And in the process,
the health professions will come to scrutinize more carefully whether
we are applying the knowledge we already have.

On Nature and Nurture

Generations of scientists and laymen have concerned themselves
with the debate over the relative primacy of heredity and environment.
In recent years the tendency has been to acknowledge the influence of
each and to focus on their interaction. It is abundantly clear that
biological organisms, no matter how well-endowed genetically, depend
upon environmental influences for their growth and development.

Much more attention has been given recently to the vulnerability
of the organism at certain periods (often referred to as "critical periods") in development. The same principles apply to psychological
and social development as to biological development. For example, it
is well known that German measles, a relatively mild disease in children, tends to produce serious abnormalities in the fetus if the mother
contracts the disease in the first third of pregnancy; or that the drug
thalidomide, which was heralded as an effective soporific with few
side-effects for adults, results in severe limb deformities in babies
when the drug is taken early in pregnancy. Older people are more
vulnerable to the respiratory hazards of air pollution. From animal
studies we know that animals reared in darkness have visual handi-

caps; and that if they do not have early, appropriate social relationships their later behavior is abnormal. These are not new concerns or observations.

Our increasing knowledge of genetics and environmental influences is destined to create new complexities. But these complexities are probably no greater than those which faced medical scientists embarking on the study of disease a century ago. Warren Weaver has stated the challenge as follows:

> These problems—and a wide range of similar problems in the biological, medical, psychological, economic and political sciences—are just too complicated to yield to the old nineteenth-century techniques which were so drastically successful on two, three, or four variable problems of simplicity. These new problems, however, cannot be handled with the statistical techniques so effective in describing average behavior in problems of disorganized complexity. These new problems—and the future of the world depends on many of them—require science to take a third great advance, an advance that must be even greater than the nineteenth-century conquest of problems of simplicity or the twentieth-century victory over problems of disorganized complexity. Science must, over the next 50 years, learn to deal with these problems of organized complexity.

In recent years there has been a growing interest in health maintenance, in contrast to the traditional focus on disease and disease prevention. There are those in medicine who feel that this is an inappropriate emphasis which need not be a concern of physicians or that health maintenance will flow logically from a continuing emphasis on the study of the nature of disease. But such matters as the application of our newer knowledge of genetics in prevention of disease, the role of family planning on health maintenance, developing early criteria for the prediction (and perhaps prevention) of disease, and the establishment of healthier environments (air, water, housing and psychological and social environments) may be developed more fully in a *health* as well as disease-oriented context.

On Minimizing Handicapping Conditions

Although precise figures are not available on the number and variety of handicapping conditions existing in school age children in this country, the Children's Bureau has estimated the prevalence of certain conditions in 1970. It is estimated that between 20 and 40 per cent of all children suffer from one or more chronic conditions (if we include eye conditions, emotional disturbances, speech problems, mental retardation, hearing impairments, and orthopedic difficulties).

Although estimates in this area are necessarily rough, it is suggested that at least a third of these handicapping conditions could be prevented, or corrected by comprehensive care prior to age six, and that continuing comprehensive care up to age eighteen would prevent or correct 60 per cent.

PRECONCEPTION

The prevention of handicapping conditions has its origins before the baby is conceived, for certain factors are associated with higher risk to the infant.

First, the physical health of the parents is of importance. Abnormalities of the genital tract, endocrine disorders of the thyroid gland, and diabetes specifically predispose to abnormalities of pregnancy and are hazards to fetal development unless carefully managed by the physician. Blood group incompatabilities between parents may predispose the fetus to certain hazards. Thus, premarital counselling should include careful physiological evaluation in addition to the provision of sexual information.

Second, the age of the parents may influence the outcome. At the two extremes of maternal age, there are distinctly greater risks of pregnancy than at the more optimal child-bearing period of the twenties and thirties. The young teen-age mother and the woman over 40 are subject to greater risks, as are their infants.

Third, family planning has implications for pregnancy outcome. The general issues of population growth and possible overpopulation will not be dealt with here. For individual families, planning is desirable with respect to genetic backgrounds, age of parents, and numbers of children. All of the variables are individual matters. Morally, it is up to each set of parents to chart its course. Professionally, a growing body of knowledge can be made available.

Numbers of children are consistently greater in low-income than in middle-income families. And if a handicapping condition is present in a child in a large family, there is a greater problem in providing appropriate care. The attitude that low-income families are not receptive to counselling regarding family size has been disproved. Once family planning information is made available to low-income population groups, the birth rate can be shown to decrease significantly. More consistent efforts must be extended to develop means of providing family planning information to as wide an audience as possible. Continuity in health services which includes family planning probably will provide the most effective long-term approach.

Fourth, genetic factors are of significance. Genetic counselling centers are now available throughout the United States for couples who have a family history of genetic abnormalities or who have had a child with an abnormality. The increase in our knowledge of such disorders has come from three main sources in recent years:

1. *Cytogenetics*—This is the science of chromosomal studies. It is now feasible (though costly) to study the numbers and shapes of chromosomes. In the past ten years many congenital abnormalities have been found to be associated with chromosomal abnormalities. Since such studies can also be done on non-affected family members, greater knowledge of possible repetition or transmission of the disorder is obtained. Now the knowledge so gained is often not a precise basis for prediction, but in the next several years will probably become much more accurate.

2. *Biochemical Genetics*—In recent years many inborn errors of metabolism such as PKU (phenylketonuria—a condition associated with mental retardation) have been studied in detail. The revolution in biology which has recently resulted in the isolation of a gene (the constituents of chromosomes) by a Harvard Medical School team headed by Dr. Jonathan Beckwith suggests that there may be some possibilities of correcting such chemical defects in genes in the future. In the meantime, dietary management in some disorders of sugar metabolism (galactosemia), amino acid metabolism (such as PKU), and other inborn errors of metabolism is helpful.

3. *Population Genetics*—As we come to know more about how abnormalities are transmitted in families, counselling can become more precise. This is an old approach, but it has added to our knowledge significantly in recent years. If family planning is to become more effective, counselling services need to be made more generally available. Low-income populations in the past have been particularly lacking in such services.

PRENATAL CARE

In any discussion of handicapping conditions, and their prevention, environmental hazards to the fetus and mother must be defined and eliminated if we are to make additional progress. The intrauterine environment is of consequence, as we have learned from the effects of drugs such as thalidomide on the fetus, and there are no guarantees that such tragedies will not recur in the future. The number of different medications taken by pregnant women in this country averages about four, and the various fetal or newborn effects of a whole series of medications are under intensive study. Intrauterine infections with syphilis, German measles virus, a parasite-toxoplasmosis, and cytomegalo-virus are some which take their toll. Preventive approaches (e.g., use of vaccines against German measles) will serve to decrease morbidity and mortality in the near future. The history of blood group incompatibility between mother and baby resulting in jaundice and possibly brain damage (erythroblastosis fetalis)—its description, etiology, treatment and now prevention, all within a single generation —should serve as a model for approaches which in the future will lead to the ultimate prevention of other diseases of the fetus and newborn, such as respiratory distress syndrome of newborn infants, and prematurity.

Other factors affecting the fetus which have been ascribed to the environment, such as X-ray radiation hazards, have been implicated in chromosomal damage. Smoking during pregnancy, urinary tract infections, malnutrition, inadequate prenatal care, and other factors have been associated with low-birth-weight infants and perhaps prematurity. With the multiplicity of factors involved in the development of birth defects and subsequent handicapping conditions, the field of genetic and conception counselling will take on a more meaningful role in the next decade. Birth defects centers in various areas of the country appropriately are adding preventive approaches to their treatment programs.

Finally, just as an optimum environment is needed for physical growth and development, it is similarly needed for favorable psychosocial development. Many observers have shown that prematurity and low birth weight of the infant are more often associated with later mental subnormality, multiple neurological handicaps, and neuropsychiatric problems than is the case in normal pregnancy. The emotional, psychological, social, and economic implications for the child and family of a child born with a handicap are formidable.

INFANT MORTALITY RATES

The health of infants in our society has improved significantly over the past several decades. In the early decades of the century, the infant mortality rate dropped precipitously from approximately 140 per 1,000 live births to approximately 22 per 1,000 in 1968.

Since 1950, however, the progress has been slower. Infant mortality rates have plateaued, and the relative position of the United States slipped to sixteenth among the countries of the world in 1968. That the rate of decline would become slower was to be expected, but no one has proposed that it should become stationary or that our relative position should decline. Some of the major factors affecting the infant mortality rate seem to be social and economic; racial factors are influenced by both.

Infant mortality rates in the nonwhite population are considerably higher than in the white population. The mortality rate for nonwhite infants between one month and one year is triple the white rate. Even more striking is the increase in the gap between the two populations over the decade since 1960. Perinatal mortality and maternal mortality rates for the nonwhite population have actually increased relative to the white. Maternal mortality rates are four times higher among nonwhites than among whites. Recent analyses of data emphasize the greater significance of economic factors over racial factors.

Such emphasis as we have placed on prevention in the past several decades has had a greater effect on the more affluent families. A study shows that infant mortality figures for the city of Baltimore, Maryland, in 1963 vary inversely with the social class, but also demonstrate the consistently higher rates for nonwhites regardless of class. The statistics on perinatal mortality in the affluent community can rival the best figures internationally.

Yerby has reported shocking differences in mortality rates in geographic subdivisions of New York City, which are pertinent. The infant mortality rate in central Harlem (a predominantly low-income nonwhite community) was 49.5 in 1962, while in Kips Bay-Yorkville (a middle-class white community about one mile away) the infant mortality rate was 14.7.

A critical evaluation of our infant health data leads us to the conclusion that we *can* provide infant care comparable in quality to that of other countries. The data suggest that further improvement in our national ranking will depend on creating a favorable prenatal and infant care environment for the low-income and the nonwhite population.

The Effects of Poverty on Physical and Mental Health

Probably the single most important factor affecting in a negative way the health of our youth is poverty in about one-quarter of the nation's children. Often indistinguishable from the problem of poverty is the high correlation of nonwhite Americans with low socioeconomic status. Nonwhite children are four times as likely as white children to be raised in economic deprivation. Thus, it is often difficult, if not impossible, to separate the two factors of race and income.

It is a generally accepted concept that with a higher level of infant mortality goes a greater vulnerability to later physical disability. We have data which indicate that the long-term effects of prematurity and newborn morbidity take a considerable toll in human potential on the survivors. Long-term studies of the detrimental effects of prematurity on physical development and psychologic and intellectual growth are frequently reported. A pediatrician and psychologist, Birch, summarizes the problem: "It appears that the nonwhite infant is subject to an excessive continuum of risk reflected at its extremes by perinatal, neonatal, and infant death, and in the survivors by a reduced functional potential."

Malnutrition

Retardation of physical growth may be the result of multiple influences, among which inadequate nutrition stands out. Reports have amply documented the problem of hunger and malnutrition in this country. That such a situation exists unfortunately has been disregarded for too long.

It has been observed that between 30 and 70 per cent of children in poverty areas suffer from some degree of iron-deficiency anemia. That this deficiency state occurs so commonly in this population group should not permit us to consider this normal. Although the effect on physical growth of mild degrees of anemia is not documented, certainly severe anemia can result in growth retardation. Few would suggest that any degree of deficiency can be regarded as beneficial for optimal learning ability and for the general energy level of the child.

The adverse effects on physical growth (and intellectual development) are less subtle with more severe anemia, the vitamin-deficiency states, and protein malnutrition which have been described in poverty areas, especially in the rural South. Studies in recent years have concentrated on psychological and social deprivation as well as undernutrition in retarding the development of the child. Obviously, it is extremely difficult to separate these factors for study.

Dr. Charles Lowe, a pediatrician serving as scientific director of the National Institute of Child Health and Human Development, in testimony before the Senate Select Committee on Nutrition and Related Human Needs, summarized the effects of malnutrition in childhood:

> The earlier malnutrition exists, the more devastatingly it impinges on growth and development.
> We now have unambiguous evidence from several sources of the following facts:
> 1. When a fetus receives inadequate nutrition in utero, the infant is born small, the placenta of his mother contains fewer cells than normal to nourish him, and his growth will be compromised;
> 2. When an infant undergoes nutritional deprivation during the first months of life, his brain fails to synthesize protein and cells at normal rates and consequently suffers a decrease as great as twenty per cent in the cell number;

3. During the last trimester of pregnancy, protein synthesis by the brain is proceeding at a very rapid rate. Immediately upon delivery, this rapid rate decreases, although it still continues at a greater pace than at later times of life. In animals, this sharp decrease in protein synthesis immediately after birth occurs in both full-term and premature animals. The decrease in protein synthesis occurring in premature animals in all probability also occurs in premature human infants. If we can extend animal observations to the human situation, we have a logical explanation for one of the most distressing concomitants of prematurity; as many as fifty per cent of prematurely born infants grow to maturity with an intellectual competence significantly below that which would be expected when compared with siblings and even age peers.

4. Severe malnutrition suffered during childhood affects learning ability, body growth, rate of maturation, ultimate size, and if prolonged, productivity.

These facts clarify our concept of the crucial importance of nutrition at certain critical times during the growth cycle of the brain and body of infants and children. The presence of malnutrition during the first five years of life constitutes a danger not only to the individual child, but also, when this exists among a significant segment of our population, to our nation as a whole.

In a study of almost 1,000 migrant children over a period of two summers in upstate New York in the early 1960s, Bergstrom found a high proportion of children had a height at or below the lower third percentile by normal standards. Twenty-five per cent of the children in the age group one to three years were in the lower third percentile by normal standards; and 13 per cent of all children fell below this level.

The grim documentation of nutritional deficiency stands as a striking counterpoint to our affluent society. What is amazing in this mass media era is the apparent lack of knowledge about such conditions outside the radius of a local community or section of the country. In certain depressed areas, such as Appalachia, in some parts of the southeastern states, and on some Indian reservations, malnutrition is similar to that found in certain developing nations of the world. Our expressions of concern for developing nations must sound hollow indeed when we are unable to feed adequately our own population. The 1969 White House Conference on Food, Nutrition, and Health made many recommendations for the correction of this inadequacy.

Dental Health

Dental abnormalities—including dental caries—constitute the most common health problem of children and adults. The onset is usually in early childhood with poor diet, poor oral hygiene, and often failure to receive prompt and adequate dental care. An estimated 20 per cent of all adults are completely without teeth, and in almost 100 million others at least half their teeth are either decayed, missing, or filled. These findings are particularly apparent in the Selective Service examinations of young adults. The prevalence of the problem is greater in families of low income.

The National Health Survey found that about 50 per cent of all children under age fifteen never have visited a dentist. In a survey of presumably normal high school students in a suburb of Pittsburgh, at least 30 per cent were found to have significant (referable) dental problems, including severe caries ("two or more teeth, largely destroyed by caries and unrepaired") and orthodontic abnormalities. The rate of severe caries increased with advancing age, and it was interesting to note that severe dental caries were associated with poor academic achievement and high absence frequency.

The child living in poverty is much less likely to receive dental care than his more affluent peers. In 1963, for example, 60 per cent of children whose family income was less than $2,000 had never been to a dentist, as compared to 10 per cent of those whose family income was over $7,000. In the summer of 1966, only one in four children examined in Project Headstart programs had ever been to a dentist, and between 40 and 90 per cent of the children examined had dental caries (depending on whether drinking water was fluoridated). Despite the fact that restorative dentistry is now accepted as an essential aspect of dental care for children, the child of poverty is much more likely to be treated by extractions rather than the filling of cavities, when he does receive care.

The implications of fluoridated water supplies in prevention of caries are now clear, although the difficulties of obtaining acceptance of fluoridation in various places are well known. Community water fluoridation reduces the cost of dental care for children by reducing the hazard of tooth loss as well as by keeping the cost of annual treatment at a level which makes it feasible for individual families and the community to maintain dental health.

Although a serious shortage of dentists prevails, early and continuing care might conserve manpower in the long run. Approaches to the training and utilization of dental health assistants have shown such technicians to be effective in the performance of many procedures. The American Dental Association has had more foresight than many other professional organizations in its advocacy of a national program for dental health. Unfortunately, relatively little has been done to implement its recommendations. We have enough knowledge to prevent or to correct most of the dental disease which develops in our young population.

Early Social and Psychological Development

Personality development is closely associated with the educational process as well as with family and community living. In recent years we have come to appreciate more fully the relationships between intellectual and personality development. When we consider that greater cognitive capacities increase the capacity for adaptation and that mental health enhances intellectual potentialities, it is clear that the approaches of the psychologist Piaget (who has studied patterns of learning) and Freud (who studied the development of personality) are not unrelated. Since the child's main task during childhood is learning, it is desirable that he have the opportunity for optimal emotional, psychological and social growth and adaptation. This process starts in early infancy with warm family relationships, extends through childhood with limit-setting by a responsible adult (parent) and society (school), and continues into adolescence.

Early patterns of mothering in low-income families may differ from middle-class patterns; absence of a permanent male adult in many households is implicated as leading to difficulty in establishing a masculine identity in many boys growing up in poverty; the recent migration of many families from the rural South to urban ghettos has resulted in disruption of families and family ties and has complicated child-rearing styles. With this as a background, many economically deprived children feel that they face a strange and hostile environment and may react with self-doubt, passivity, and dependency, or in a violent, destructive manner, to stressful situations.

Because of the national concern over the mental health of children, Congress established in 1966 a Joint Commission on Mental Health of Children. This group has studied all aspects of the development of children and youth in America, and has made recommendations for future action and programs to provide for a more favorable environment for all our children. Many gaps in the availability of services have been identified, among which is the fact that in most communities mental health facilities for children—particularly low-income children—are sorely lacking.

The Need for Early Learning

Abundant data illustrate the developmental decline which takes place in young children of low-income background. Deutsch has indicated that by the time of school age, the discrepancy in performance of this group of children increases rather than diminishes. Although the developmental consequences of depriving environments have been described in quantitative terms, a good general description has been written by Wortis and her colleagues in the concluding paragraph of a study of child-rearing practices with 250 prematurely born infants:

> Other elements than the child-rearing patterns in the environment were preparing the child to take over a lower-class role. The inadequate incomes, crowded homes, lack of consistent family ties, the mother's depression and helplessness in her own situation, were as important as her child-rearing practices in influencing the child's development and preparing him for an adult role. It was for us a sobering experience to watch a large group of newborn infants, plastic human beings of unknown potential, and observe over a five-year period their social preparation to enter the class of the least-skilled, least-educated, and most-rejected in our society.

It is, of course, inappropriate to assume that all children are equally vulnerable to depriving environments or that this process develops uniformly. In our studies the decline is observed to start by one year of age. Bayley has demonstrated no significant differences on the basis of social class up to fifteen months of age. But all studies dealing with deprived and nondeprived preschool or kindergarten children show, by three years of age, a deficit in functioning levels of the deprived groups.

Our knowledge of the impact of depriving environments on early development has accumulated over recent years. The pediatric, psychiatric, psychological, and social work literature has recorded the unfortunate effects of depriving environments in young children living in institutions. Perhaps it was the clinical orientation of this literature and its focus on institutions which blinded us to the more subtle aspects of the effects of environmental deprivation on large numbers of children living with their families.

Some of the current enrichment programs are attempting to deal with the early manifestations of environmental deprivation. These experiences suggest that the optimal time for trying to minimize or reverse the effects of deprivation is during the early years when the children are seldom under systematic observation by professional groups and services.

The enrichment programs for infants currently in progress are varied. Some utilize day care programs as well as parental involvement. Others emphasize home visits and "tutoring" (we have not yet developed a good vocabulary for these programs) of infants. These programs are showing that given the appropriate circumstances (physical environment, personnel, and program), day care can stimulate intellectual, emotional, and social development in children whose families and/or home environments might not be able to provide such stimulation.

As these research programs attain greater maturity we will have some much needed information about the long-term effects of enrichment upon the cognitive, social, and emotional development of infants. In the process we will learn much more about "optimal" environments for infants and young children. These programs are directing attention to the possibilities of a national program. It is essential, if we are to move in that direction, to insure the quality of care and to avoid the unfortunate effects of custodial group care of infants and young children which were so prevalent in the past.

The Need for Programs

Our society has made a basic value judgment concerning the importance of education. As a consequence school attendance is compulsory. Even with all our problems concerning the quality of education, the wisdom of this decision still stands. It is now well known that many children from economically deprived populations reach school age unprepared to benefit from our educational system. Until recently, emphasis has been placed on remedial or compensatory programs for school children of all ages, once a problem is identified within the system. We have had enough experience to know that in spite of heroic efforts, these programs have not produced a positive yield. As in medicine generally, prevention would seem to be a more rational and humanitarian approach.

In recognition of this problem, the Office of Economic Opportunity —established by the Economic Opportunity Act of 1964, which was passed as a consequence of the civil rights movement and the growing concern for the poor—initiated Project Headstart for preschool children. The introduction of the report of the Planning Committee for Project Headstart given to President Johnson in February 1965 presented the problem as follows:

> There is considerable evidence that the early years of childhood are the most critical point in the poverty cycle. During these years the creation

of learning patterns, emotional development and the formation of individual expectations and aspirations take place at a very rapid pace. For the child of poverty there are clearly observable deficiencies in the processes which lay the foundation for a pattern of failure—and thus a pattern of poverty—throughout the child's entire life.

Within recent years there has been experimentation and research designed to improve opportunities for the child of poverty. While much of this work is not yet complete there is adequate evidence to support the view that special programs can be devised for these four and five year olds which will improve both the child's opportunities and achievements. It is clear that successful programs of this type must be comprehensive, involving activities generally associated with the fields of health, social services, and education. Similarly it is clear that the program must focus on the problems of child and parent and that these activities need to be carefully integrated with programs for the school years.

We frequently refer to our children as our greatest natural resource, yet our efforts to develop this resource fully have been sorely lacking. The data derived from the Headstart program demonstrated major gaps in health care for children approaching school age who grow up in economically deprived homes. If the main "task" of childhood is learning, one can assume a child will be less adequately equipped to perform his task if he does not have optimum sensory capacity—particularly in vision and hearing—and optimum health. Without intervention at the time of the Headstart program, these children would presumably begin their formal educational experience with significant physiological handicaps.

It has now been clearly demonstrated that an intervention program can favorably affect the ability of children to develop intellectually. There has been appropriate concern that children participating in summer enrichment programs may lose many of the developmental gains when enrolled into a continuing school environment which fails to provide ongoing adequate stimulation. Thus, considerable effort must be placed on developing follow-through programs in the public school system. It may well be that in the long perspective, one of the main contributions of Headstart will have been its impact on improving the quality of education in the elementary grades.

Just as follow-through is important, earlier intervention or prevention prior to the Headstart years (three to five years) may be of even greater importance. Day care programs for younger children have been acceptable means of providing for the developmental needs of communities of children in Russia, Israel, and other countries, for some time. In this country, emphasis has been placed on the value of individual care in the family, and we have tended to steer away from group programs for young children. Several factors now make for urgent reevaluation of these concepts in America. Among them are the transplantation of approximately 100,000 people per year in the post World War II period from environments of rural poverty to those of urban poverty, complicating the problem of family life and child care in the city; and the intense pressure by society on mothers in single-parent families to return to educational and training programs or to employment. This pressure, by the way, reverses an approach instituted almost 40 years ago when the value judgment was made that it was better for young children to have their mothers at home—one of the basic premises of the Aid to Dependent Children Program initiated in the 1930s.

The School Years

The psychoanalyst Erikson has defined the developmental task of the school age child as the development of a sense of industry. This develops out of play which becomes more complex as the child grows older, and involves preparation for adult living through learning to live by "rules of the game." Also, a sense of industry stems from the engagement with learning tasks in the group setting of the school.

The physical problems of the child must be taken into account in planning his educational program. In recent decades the schools have developed special programs for children with specific handicaps. Since it is estimated that more than five million children are in need of special education, the provision of adequate resources and manpower is proving a formidable challenge for school districts and colleges of education.

During the school years, emotional problems which have gone unrecognized or unattended often become apparent. The National Institute of Mental Health, on the basis of various school surveys, estimated that 1,400,000 children under eighteen years needed psychiatric treatment in 1966. Unfortunately many of these children are ultimately excluded from school and become social and psychiatric problems of the community.

Since our society has a universal requirement of school attendance, the inadequate academic achievement of children readily becomes apparent. The emphasis on educational achievement in recent years (stimulated in no small measure by the Russians' launching of the Sputniks) has highlighted our failures and resulted in programs of compensatory or remedial education, particularly for children of low-income families.

As indicated earlier, much stress has been placed in recent years on the various factors leading to psychological deprivation and intellectual retardation. We have commented on the phenomenon of retardation on the basis of suboptimal intra-uterine environment, prematurity and perinatal morbidity, as well as some of the factors associated with economic deprivation, such as poor nutrition and ill health. These factors will account for some of the poor performance of children of low-income families in the American school system.

In addition, we now have data to suggest that many of the children from deprived backgrounds are virtually "programmed" for failure. Studies have shown that some ghetto children, rather than growing up in an environment of sensory deprivation, actually are exposed to excessive or inappropriate stimulation and may have learned to "tune-out" much of the background noise of their environments. Thus, they may tend to tune-out the teacher and *appropriate* stimulation in the classroom. If the child is in a class with children from varied backgrounds, he may readily fall farther behind as the rest of the class progresses. Given a majority of pupils in the class with similar backgrounds, it is not difficult to see how the entire class would have difficulty progressing. Such are the problems faced by children attending the neighborhood school in the ghettos of our cities.

Among all economic groups, learning disorders, as defined by poor school achievement, are common. It is estimated that ten per cent of children experience such problems. The causes range from psychological difficulties to brain dysfunction and are often mixed in origin.

In recent years considerable attention has been directed to so-called minimal cerebral dysfunction or "brain damage." Some of these children, on retrospective history, present evidence of having had a difficult time at labor and/or delivery (either too rapid or prolonged) leading to asphyxia and presumably to the syndrome of hyperactivity, short attention span, reading disability, and other specific learning disorders. This particular group of findings also seems to occur more frequently among children born in low-income families, since it would appear to be related to perinatal morbidity. Perinatal morbidity, like mortality, is significantly greater in the nonwhite than white population, and in the lower than in upper socioeconomic population. Children with "brain damage," once identified, may be amenable to treatment with drugs to decrease their hyperactivity and in some school systems are provided special programs to fit their needs—small classes, and intensive efforts by specially trained therapists and instructors.

The great majority of our school systems at the present time are not equipped to identify adequately the various problems leading to intellectual retardation. The poorer the neighborhood school and the larger the classes, the less likely are individual problems to be recognized early, and even when recognized, the less likely are there to be facilities or personnel to manage these problems optimally. The continuation of a child needing special treatment within the educational system, without adequate professional help, serves as a source of considerable difficulty for the teacher, the school, the child and his peers. Thus, children from economically deprived families are often trapped in classroom situations with children manifesting heterogeneous learning disorders ranging from the moderately retarded to the emotionally disturbed, with all variations between. Even the child who is highly motivated can scarcely be expected to reach his greatest potentiality in such an educational milieu. Attention is being directed to developing more adequate, comprehensive mental health programs, along with general health services, for school age children.

Adolescence

Adolescence is usually defined as the state or process of growing up from childhood to manhood or womanhood. This is a relatively long period of years characterized by striking biological, psychological, and social changes. The rate at which these changes take place is dramatic and the complexity of the changes causes many observers to wonder about why so much "goes right" rather than why so much "goes wrong" in adolescence.

Individual differences become strikingly apparent during adolescence. Variations in the onset of biological growth and the concomitant sexual maturation create an accentuation of differences. The two sexes differ in the time of onset of changes; girls generally mature biologically approximately two years earlier than boys. The control mechanism for initiating the changes in growth is not well understood. It would appear to be under genetic influence from centers in the brain, which act in concert with the pituitary gland at the base of the brain which in turn regulates growth and many metabolic processes in the body.

That the genetically regulated growth processes of adolescence are subject to environmental influences is evident from the earlier onset of these changes which has been taking place in recent decades. Biological adolescence begins approximately four years earlier than it did a century and a half ago. This is probably due to improvement in nutrition and general health, although it would seem reasonable to believe that this trend will level off.

The growth and developmental changes may be understood more clearly if they are classified about the central events of rapid growth and the attainment of sexual maturity (pubescence). In the female the onset of menstruation marks pubescence; in the male this is not so clearly defined, but rapid genital growth and the appearance of mature pubic hair are comparable events.

PREPUBESCENCE

Prepubescence is characterized by the initiation of more rapid growth and by the early manifestations of secondary sexual characteristics (development of voice changes, growth of beard, and pubic hair in males; the rounding of hips, budding of breasts, and appearance of pubic hair in girls). Since these changes occur at rather widely varying ages, children of the same chronological age may have very different maturational states and feelings; school programs should take these factors into account even though it is difficult in a group setting to individualize programs for individual children.

The most rapid physical growth occurs in the period just prior to the onset of pubescence. There may be a gain of 7 to 8 inches in height and 20 to 30 pounds in weight during a year. It is small wonder that the adolescent may appear to be awkward (although objective tests of coordination do not confirm that the adolescent is truly awkward; indeed, he usually is very well-coordinated in his performance of such tests and in athletics).

This rapid growth with accompanying primary and secondary sexual characteristics of adolescent boys and girls suggests that they must develop new relationships (or perceptions) of their bodies. The prepubescent period, therefore, is one in which there is often considerable anxiety concerning feelings of inadequacy or inferiority. The opportunity to gain reassurance through a physical examination by a physician is extremely important. Anxiety concerning sexual adequacy or inadequacy of knowledge may cause discomfort. The perceptive physician, through his skillful physical examination, may relieve such anxiety and he may also utilize the opportunity to provide factual information concerning sexual development.

The anxiety concerning anticipated sexual changes suggests the need for sex education for school children. Factual knowledge can help each child deal with his feelings. Although there has been controversy concerning the introduction of sex education in the schools, it would seem desirable to provide—in ways appropriate for the child's age—an adequate background of knowledge. While the home is the primary base for providing such knowledge and attitudes, the schools can play an important role in the development of an adequate vocabulary and information. If such knowledge is not forthcoming, the child has haphazardly acquired information and his fantasies to rely upon, which may accentuate the anxiety.

The psychological stresses of this period probably result in variations in school performance or psychosomatic disorders. Thus, refusal to eat (anorexia nervosa) may occur and such disorders as obesity, ulcerative colitis, peptic ulcer, and early manifestations of high blood pressure may also develop. The precise way in which these disorders are caused by the subtle (often unconscious) anticipation of sexual maturation is not known. Often there is a clustering of stresses possibly related to school performance, emotional difficulties within the family, separation from a close friend or relative, or other traumatic situations which together produce such reactions.

POSTPUBESCENCE

The period following pubescence is that generally referred to in popular literature as adolescence. Chronologically, depending on the age of the development of sexual maturity, this period has its onset from twelve to fourteen years—earlier for girls than for boys and with a considerable range for each sex. During this period the adaptation of the child to his or her bodily changes and new contours continues.

Disorders—The biological changes and stresses predispose to various disorders. Thyroid gland disturbances may occur; this gland is very involved in the hormonal changes going on normally. A tendency to obesity may develop, especially in girls; although there may be a genetic predisposition, inappropriate diet and/or excessive eating is a more usual cause. Since overeating usually has some psychological basis, the cause of psychological difficulties probably needs to be defined. Acne is a common concomitant of hormonal changes in adolescence. Its severity varies widely and medical advice concerning its care is desirable, since self-medication may aggravate the condition. It is unfortunate that this skin problem occurs at this time, since it is during this period that the child's mental capacity has matured to the point at which he begins to "see himself as others see him." The presence of acne may reinforce feelings of inadequacy or inferiority which are so common during this time.

Psychological Development—The psychological and social developmental tasks of adolescence are a major concern of our society. Each generation of parents tends to feel that current adolescents are the most difficult. Whether the earlier biological onset of growth and maturational changes, the tendency for prolongation of economic dependence through extension of collegiate education and graduate and professional education, and the rapid communication of the mass media have indeed made adolescence more complicated and stressful, it is difficult to say. Also, the adult world for which the adolescent is preparing is more complex. But the basic tasks of psychological development remain the same over the generations. The British psychoanalyst Winnicott states:

> I constantly remind myself that it is the state of adolescence that society perpetually carries, not the adolescent boy or girl who, alas, in a few years becomes adult, and who becomes only too soon identified with some kind of frame in which new babies, new children, and new adolescents may be free to have vision and dreams and new plans for the world. Triumph belongs to the attainment of maturity by growth process. Triumph does not belong to the false maturity based on a facile impersonation of an adult.

The psychological tasks of the adolescent revolve around the establishment of a sense of identity. All past experiences and significant relationships must be integrated in developing a feeling about "who-ness and what-ness" for each person. A sense of identity involves bringing together many factors related to sexual identification, nationality (often rendered more difficult in a country like the United States with people of heterogeneous backgrounds), religion, education, economic, racial and social background, and occupation of parents. The process of incorporating what has gone before with what the adolescent aspires to be is complex. But the past cannot be denied; out-of-sight is not out-of-mind. The adolescent who is trying to run away from his heritage will find difficulty in later adjustment.

Autonomy—Another developmental task is that of increasing autonomy. In preparation for the more adult role of leaving home to establish a career and possibly a new family, the adolescent needs opportunities for increasing autonomy. Summer camp, college attendance, and work experience provide some such opportunities. Autonomy is also manifested ideologically; declarations of independence may be made visible by embracing ideologies at variance with, or in opposition to, parental values and standards. The rebellion of youth can be understood better in this context. It is to be emphasized that capacities for abstract thinking become well-developed during this age period; for the first time concepts such as justice, charity, sympathy, and pity have meaning and are being explored. Adolescents, singly and in groups, with idealistic motivation challenge society for its incapacity to solve its social problems. Group confrontations may be stimulated by the presence of serious social, economic, and racial problems in the presence of long continued affluence and great productive capacity. The translation of these idealistic aspirations into continuing constructive programs for social change is one of the central problems of our society—not alone that of adolescents and young adults. The mass media, particularly television, may play significant roles in the epidemiology of rebellion and confrontation. In contrast to the pre-television era, the techniques of one group may become known almost instantaneously to other groups and applied, whether the issues are the same or not.

An affiliation with a group—in ideology, dress, or tastes in music—is often employed by adolescents in facilitating the separation from the family. Parents have difficulty in accepting this transition, since the group may have values in conflict with those of the family. It is possible to understand the meaning of such group affiliations in the light of the background of the individual adolescent.

The psychoanalyst Erikson has defined the adolescent mind as "essentially a mind of the moratorium, a psychosocial stage . . . between the morality learned by the child, and the ethics to be developed by the adult." If this transition becomes too difficult the moratorium might become pronounced with the individual dropping out of school or society generally. This is not a new phenomenon, but again the epidemiology may be different now. The use of drugs is another way of dropping out, if carried to extremes. This is a period of experimentation with various life styles and often re-entry into the mainstream of society takes place if it is not made too difficult.

Heterosexual Relationships—Another developmental task for the adolescent is the establishment of heterosexual relationships. The capacity for a more mature sexual role is a reflection of all prior life experiences. Social relationships may be fostered by well-planned activities for adolescents.

Complexity of Growth—The complexity of biological, phschological, and social growth during this period is not always completely balanced and integrated. For example, a boy of fifteen years of age may be biologically at the thirteen-year level, seventeen years intellectually, and fifteen psychologically. How old is he? During this period various emotional difficulties may become apparent. High anxiety levels may interfere with learning, feelings of inferiority may interfere with social adjustment and school achievements, and feelings of despair and worthlessness may result in suicidal thoughts or acts. Rebelliousness or other problems may stimulate delinquent behavior. Occasionally psychosomatic symptoms occur. And if the stress is unduly great or there is predisposition, disorganization of personality in the form of psychosis may occur. For adolescence is the summing up; if early experiences and the adolescent years have not prepared the person for impending adult life, emotional disturbance is the result.

School Drop-Outs—We have described previously some of the factors affecting the child from low socioeconomic families resulting in the situation where he starts school behind his age-mates, and drops farther behind with each passing year. As he progresses through the school system, frequently passed on by the single criterion of advancing chronologic age, he reaches adolescence often barely literate. He thus becomes a "drop-out" as he reaches the mandated age of sixteen. The system has been unable to cope with the student's problems, and after spending eleven or twelve years within the school system, he leaves virtually unprepared for any but the most menial of jobs, and with little prospects for the future.

Certainly many factors are involved in this phenomenon. Among these should be mentioned the parental loss of initiative and motivation for learning. Children whose parents have lost hope for the future, who have been passive recipients of economic assistance for one or two generations, and who have no prospects for change in their own lives, can also be expected to have little motivation. In placing a high premium on college education, we have not provided for adequate alternative routes for those students not going on for further education.

Adolescent Goals—The adolescent from a privileged home has various alternatives (college education, employment, etc.) which the child from a low-income home often does not have. In a society affluent for a long period of years, many adolescents have difficulty in identifying clear goals. Meaningful work opportunity which provides outlets for the idealistic aspirations of youth (such as Peace Corps, VISTA, Headstart, etc.) may help in the mastery of difficulties associated with the transition to adult life. In some societies where adolescents are relied upon for meaningful work and where goals are clearly defined (Israel, for example), there is relatively little of the adolescent unrest described elsewhere.

Manpower Development—The Job Corps Program of the Office of Economic Opportunity, initiated in 1965, is an example of an attempt to intervene in the cycle leading to intellectual and functional wastage among the youth of the lower socioeconomic population. That this program has been the target of much criticism is perhaps symbolic of a general feeling of frustration with remedial programs at all levels. The successes of the Job Corps and other manpower development programs should not be ignored. Although we are committed to the ideal of prevention, we must not forget that at least for some time to come, we are also committed to compensating for the gaps of the past.

Unmarried Pregnant Adolescent—Another example of a remedial approach is noted in programs directed toward the unmarried pregnant adolescent. A significant number of teenage pregnancies occur among low-income families, although there is some evidence to suggest that out-of-wedlock pregnancies in adolescents have increased over the past several years, in general. Among the girls from low-income families, the alternatives are strictly limited. Short of obtaining an illegal abortion, the girl has little choice but to continue with the pregnancy, and she or her mother keeps the infant in the family. Private sources of institutional care for the pregnant girl are few and are limited by expense to the upper socioeconomic population. Facilities for adoption, and/or foster care, for the infant are difficult to obtain for the lower socioeconomic population, particularly for the nonwhites. Thus, the low-income/poor-health cycle is perpetuated. The hazards of pregnancy for mother and baby in the early teen years has stimulated much effort to reform the abortion laws to make the procedure legal if it is sought.

Historically in the educational system, being pregnant was the surest way for a girl to be expelled from school. More recently, however, some communities have taken significant steps in an attempt to maintain the girl's educational programs, and to restore opportunity for further education or better employment. Pregnant adolescents in some of these programs are brought together in a formal school setting which also includes intensive contacts with psychologists, social service personnel, and health professionals. In many of these girls significant psychological problems may be present, either as cause for the pregnancy or as a complication of it. The girls continue their education without interruption through pregnancy and return to school as soon as they are physically able after delivery.

Despite these significant remedial programs, we must sound a cautionary note: in the long run, programs designed toward prevention must have a more significant yield in terms of salvage rates of our adolescent population. We must consider the impact on the adolescent girl, her family, and the offspring of the out-of-wedlock pregnancies. There are explorations of programs for the dissemination of family planning information for young people in order to create a better-informed generation which will be oriented toward the planning for children and thereby minimize the occurrence of unwanted pregnancies. Also, programs of education for family living are being explored in many schools. Although some people oppose such instruction on the basis that it dilutes the intellectual content of the curriculum, there is no reason to believe that the teaching of reproduction and human relationships needs to be lacking in intellectual content or mental stimulation.

Early Adult Years (Ages 20 to 30)

In our culture the end point of adolescence is not clearly defined. The prolongation of higher education often fosters economic dependency even when biological and social maturity have developed. Such dependency complicates courting and marriage and places pressures on parents to continue some measure of financial support for their children even after they have married. Young adults enrolled in professional educational programs such as medicine may not become economically self-sufficient until their late twenties.

This is a period of relatively good physical health. Medical care generally centers about intercurrent illnesses such as acute respiratory infections. Obstetrical care also is a stimulus for general medical care. Although there may be relatively little physical illness, this is a period in which sound, regular patterns of medical care should be established. Counselling concerning exercise and recreation, diet, drinking and smoking, and work habits can be helpful to the young adult in establishing a constructive life style.

Freud, when asked what he thought a normal person should be able to do well, responded simply by saying: "To love and to work." These are the central developmental tasks of the young adult. The patterns of courting, marriage (or lack of it), and childbearing are reflections of the culture in which young adults were reared and now live. The complexity of developing patterns of heterosexual intimacy is such that separation and divorce have become relatively common. Many value judgments are made concerning divorce rates; an optimistic interpretation may be that such separations represent constructive efforts at adjustment.

The mobility of our population is such that many young adults are at considerable distance from their parents and grandparents, in contrast to other cultures in which there is more geographic stability and ethnic homogeneity. Under these circumstances, young families tend to turn to professional services and agencies for help and counselling which was previously provided within the family. Professionals in medicine, social work, and psychology need a sound background in helping people to adapt to new experiences through premarital and family planning counselling, pregnancy, infant and child care, and emotional stresses.

Health and social agencies can be particularly helpful with child-rearing problems in "one-parent families." In instances of emotional crisis such as in separation or divorce, professional services may be extremely helpful. Also in low-income populations, welfare programs in the past have often discouraged marriages (through deprivation of assistance if there is "a man in the house"). Planning for day care for young children as desired may be helpful in the adaptation of parents and children to adverse circumstances. In the past, group care for young children was in disfavor among professionals because of the custodial nature of such care. There is now considerable emphasis on the provision of stimulating, intimate caretaking for the child and also on the involvement of parents in the program.

The establishment of a work career and earning capacity is another of the adaptations to be made. A large group of young people traverse this period having acquired their desired education and skills and are in pursuit of relatively clear goals. Some young people from affluent circumstances experience a continuation of the psychosocial moratorium of adolescence, have no clear goals or motivation, and are diffuse in their activities. It is not clear whether the number of such young people is increasing; their presence is more apparent to society. Another group of young people who have difficulty in entering productive work careers are those of low economic background who have been unable to take advantage of earlier educational experiences in order to develop a vocational background. Recent programs by government and industry designed to prepare such young people for work are having some constructive impact. These programs deserve a high priority, for the alternative is despair and often antisocial behavior.

A note is in order on the role of the young woman. If she is married she often feels unprepared for a role as homemaker and mother. The transition from school or work may be difficult; she may feel trapped or bored. The possible combination of work or community activities may help in the transition. Again, adequate child care facilities may be very helpful. For low-income mothers, often alone and with little relief from child care activities, there may be strong feelings of hopelessness and helplessness which unfortunately are readily perceived by children. Child care facilities may be helpful not only in providing some relief and assistance, but also in combining part-time education and vocational preparation for those who are interested in work.

The Middle Years (Ages 30 to 65)

The middle years of life are generally the peak period of work productivity and concern with family life and the rearing of children.

Because of its significance to society and the span of years it occupies, it is surprising that it has received so little attention in the professional literature. The medical literature is concerned largely with disease processes in this age period; there have been few studies of how adults cope with such crises as illness and death of parents, illness and, rarely, death of children, severe illnesses and injuries in adult life, the necessity for periodic moves to a new environment, menopausal changes, declining work productivity and impending retirement, rapid technological and social change, and movement of children away from home and marriage.

It is understandable that the health professions, by tradition and lack of adequate manpower resources, would focus on disease. But thereby they neglect to study the basis of competence, the coping ability of people, and the mastery of adversity. In recent years the armed services and industry, concerned with developing officer and executive talent, have begun to study the ingredients for successful living and performance. It has been suggested by some that, since pediatrics and geriatrics are concerned with health and medical care of children and older people, respectively, the term "mediatrics" be employed comparably for the health supervision in the middle years. It is certainly surprising to find how little literature on the growth and development of children is associated with studies of parents concurrently, since the parents are the most significant influence in the lives of their children.

During the middle years, medical care assumes a more definite place. This is the age at which tumors may begin to manifest themselves more frequently. Regular physical examinations provide opportunities for early detection and prompt treatment. Also, especially for males, the hazards of coronary artery disease become greater. Although we lack as much knowledge as we would like concerning prevention, it appears that a clustering of predisposing or causative factors is at work. In addition to genetic predisposition, the following factors seem to be of significance in causation: obesity, tendency to diabetes, high cholesterol diet, smoking, lack of exercise, and psychological stress. Since these factors are modifiable, we may have considerable potentiality for reversing the trend toward early heart attacks.

It would appear that attempts to motivate young people to establish sound health habits are in order. The 1969 White House Conference on Food, Nutrition and Health emphasized that, as an affluent nation, many people suffer from malnutrition while many others suffer from undernutrition. The average body weight has increased over the last 30 years as physical demands have dropped; simultaneously, food consumption is stimulated by advertising and higher income. Obesity also predisposes to the development of diabetes, thus increasing its hazard. Smoking also has been stimulated by advertising; efforts to discourage adolescents and adults from smoking are not well-developed as yet. The menopause as a process is unique to the human organism. Just as with adolescence, its onset is regulated by higher centers. The process is not well understood, but many of the associated hormonal changes have been studied. The process need not be accompanied by the profound biological and psychological changes once ascribed to it; physicians can do much to relieve the physiological changes. And the psychological changes can be ameliorated by an understanding that one can continue to function effectively in society. Interests in work or community activities can be very helpful in the transition. Occasionally, depressive reactions may occur in response to the menopause. Feelings of loss of self-esteem and adequacy in reaction to bodily changes may be at the basis for such disorders. The physician can usually provide help in dealing with the problem and gaining relief from it.

Depressive reactions are not uncommon in males, also, during this period. Episodes of loss of a loved person or situations in which there may be a blow to one's self-esteem, bodily injuries or illnesses, or changes in role or reductions in work capacity may precipitate such events. Sometimes these reactions are mild and manifested only by a lowering of mood or sadness, a slowing of thought processes and motor activity such as poor muscle tone and slowness in walking, or loss of appetite, or insomnia. Recognition of mild reactions may occur only by the physician through periodic examinations and evaluations. Many industries have inaugurated periodic health evaluation programs for employees in order to detect disorders early and to maintain good health.

Modern, predominantly urban, society has increased the complexity of living. Modern man in middle years needs to find ways of controlling and accommodating to the rapid pace, crowding, travel, noise, and tendency toward impersonalization and alienation if he is to gain pleasure as well as affluence.

The Later Adult Years (Ages Beyond 65)

Advances in medical knowledge have been associated with the rising number of older people in the population. In 1900, the median age of the population was 22.9 years; at that time there were 3 million people 65 years of age and older who represented 4 per cent of the total population. Sixty years later the median age was 29.5 years and there were 17 million people or 9.3 per cent of the population 65 years of age and older. In 1900 the average expectation of life at birth was 49 years; in 1964 it had become 70.2 years.

The estimated total population of the United States at the beginning of 1967 was slightly more than 198 million, of whom about 18.5 million were 65 years of age or older. The projected total population for 1975 is 230 million with some 23 million in the older age group. The increase in the proportion of older people will be only 0.5 per cent, specifically a rise to 10 per cent. Thus, it would appear that there is a leveling off of the percentage of older people in the United States.

Following the depression of the 1930s, the age of 65 was established as a retirement age, particularly through the Social Security legislation. Many employment policies in industry, governmental agencies, and universities follow this pattern. The range and variety of factors which influence functional capacity make chronological age an unreliable predictor of the need for retirement. The problems of older people have their origins in habits and patterns of living established in earlier life; some are residual from illness in earlier years; some derive from specific genetic endowment; and many stem from complex tissue alterations inherent in the process of aging and senescence. In years gone by it was customary to repeat the aphorism that if one wanted to live a long life it was desirable to have had parents who had lived to a ripe old age. The increasing life span of our population generally indicates that longevity is considerably more complex than such straightforward genetic formulations.

As a consequence of the higher frequency with which illness occurs in this age group and the gradual loss of function, available medical and social services are utilized to an increasing extent. Not only are more physician visits required per year, but the number of days of confinement to bed because of disability per year are about two and a half times greater in those above 65 than in adults below that age. Unfortunately, while the need for services is intensified, the availability of such services is often limited. Data from the National Center for Health Statistics indicate that 80 per cent of people 65 years and over have one or more chronic conditions associated with limitation of activity.

It would seem that the process of aging is inexorable and that a gradual decline in the capacity of the various body systems (respiratory, alimentary, cardiovascular, genitourinary, endocrine, musculo-skeletal, and nervous) goes on in all individuals, although at somewhat different rates for each; however, it is also apparent that the aging person usually dies from some clear-cut pathological process for which controls might potentially be developed. Thus it would seem that this is an important area for study in the older population which would be comparable to the growth and developmental types of studies in the young population. The studies of aging, however, involve the study of declining rather than growing functions.

Perhaps no period of life requires such a spectrum of services and resources as that of the older group of our population. Physicians, nurses and social workers are key personnel in the provision of health programs for the elderly. All of the allied health professions, community planners, and legislative groups are instrumental in making appropriate resources available. Unfortunately, general hospitals are too frequently the main resources available for long-term care. For long-term care, the individual without a family may require nursing home, foster home, or some other institutional care which is appropriate to meet his needs. For the patient who does have a family to care for him, several types of home care patient programs have been developed. These employ visiting nurses, homemaker services, and occasionally the provision of food services in the home. Volunteer efforts to provide personal contact and recreation can also be useful in maintaining the interest of the older person in the world about him.

The enactment of Medicare and Medicaid legislation in 1965 has helped to finance health services for those over 65 years of age. However, some of the provisions remain inadequate. The payment for medical fees is on a voluntary basis, a pattern which poses serious problems for those in precarious economic circumstances. Also the provision of funds through Medicare has not always been matched by the appropriate availability of services. Communities are being pressed to manifest more resourcefulness in the provision of a broad spectrum of services to meet the needs of the older population.

The older person is subject to all of the psychiatric difficulties of younger individuals; in addition there may be some vascular changes in the brain which might impair function. Many older people withstand vascular changes, such as multiple small strokes, with considerable resiliency and regain their cerebral and emotional functioning. However, it is difficult to determine how much psychiatric disorder may be attributable to organic changes and how much to psychological difficulties. Certainly it is recognized increasingly that many older people maintain a high order of psychological function well into old age. Enforced idleness and isolation are particularly difficult for the older person; when cut off from contact with family members, a more rapid mental and emotional decline may be observed. A tendency toward depression because of loss of physiologic function, physical inadequacy, and loss of close friends and relatives is more frequent in the older patient. The perspective on life of older patients is usually such that it is gratifying to professionals to work with them. There is deep appreciation for even symptomatic relief, and the contact with people who have grown wise and old can be extremely stimulating and helpful in the development of a professional philosophy towards the life cycle. Some of the perspective which comes with old age has been described by the novelist and essayist Frank Swinnerton as follows:

For me, it is a great privilege to be an octogenarian. The high fevers of life are over; and unless his facilities are badly rusted (which is not the experience of my octogenarian friends) the man of eighty-odd begins every day free from the anxieties, angers, and frustrations which beset his juniors. He is no longer love-sick; he has not to jostle with the crowds on train or street car; he has time to "stand and stare." Further satisfactions follow.

He is still richly alive; and having experienced nearly a hundred years of rich and turbulent history, sees the present in perspective, as more than a detail in the tremendous stream of time.

Separation

Psychosocial development may be viewed as a series of challenges for the mastery of separating experiences. With birth, one of the most profound of separating experiences occurs, biologically and psychologically. The biological event is sufficiently profound to be marked indelibly in the microscopic growth rings of the teeth. Psychologically, the event is of great real and symbolic significance for parents and, ultimately, the child in the form of birthday celebrations as a constant reminder of its meaning to the family.

The mastery of separation is a part of the successful passage of every stage of development. In infancy at seven or eight months of age, as vision matures and the infant has the capacity to recognize parents, he begins to manifest separation anxiety as they leave him. Losing parents for brief periods and finding them in a safe context becomes part of mastery. Peek-a-boo games provide a play opportunity to gain such mastery.

As the child learns to walk, physical separation becomes possible. As the child unknowingly walks out of sight of parents, he manifests anxiety; if the environment is safe, he learns to tolerate and enjoy his brief travels. If day care programs or nursery school attendance is possible, separation is feasible for longer periods. And with school attendance, a major separation for significant portions of the day occurs just as the child seems to have a capacity for such experience physically and emotionally—if all has gone well previously and if the school offers a comfortable environment.

In adolescence, longer periods are spent away from home, and summer camp or boarding school may provide a greater challenge. College attendance away from home is a major separation from which many young adults never return to live with the family.

Marriage constitutes a major separation, as well as union and challenge for a new intimacy in the establishment of a new family. With the birth of children, the cycle of separation is renewed and the challenge is to master these events more competently than one's own parents.

With aging, many other separating events occur. Losses of husband or wife or other close relatives are traumatic events. No matter what the cause, separation from a loved one is a blow to one's integrity. And finally, one must face a separating experience as profound as that of birth: death. The degree of comfort with which it is approached is a reflection—as formulated by the psychoanalyst Erikson—of the integrity of personality development. He states: ". . . healthy children will not fear life if their elders have integrity enough not to fear death."

The Need for a Favorable Ecology

In concluding, it is appropriate to return to an early theme: optimal human development is a result of the interaction of genetic potentialities with a favorable environment. Although modern society has achieved an increase in the length of life, a reversal of this trend may occur if man does not harness for progress the environmental changes he has wrought. The establishment in early 1970 of a President's Environmental Council is evidence of the concern over environmental threats to human development.

It is apparent that the many factors influencing physical and mental growth and health relate to the total environment, rather than to isolated variables. For example, medical care alone will not effectively reduce infant morbidity and mortality, for there are societies with relatively adequate medical care but with low income which have unfavorable rates. In subtle ways, food, housing, clothing, medical care, and physical, social and psychological stress exert an influence at all stages of development.

It becomes important, therefore, for the health professions, in cooperation with all concerned citizens, again to direct their attention to environmental improvement. This is not a new role, especially for those in the field of public health.

We are now in a crisis over the deterioration of our cities. For more than 25 years we have been witnessing a migration of more than 100,000 persons per year from rural poverty to urban poverty. There has been little restructuring of our cities to accommodate to these changes beyond a flight to the suburbs. The approaches taken in the past decades are ample witness to our failure to face the tremendous housing shortage of our urban and rural poor.

It would seem that our next creative efforts will need to be directed toward bringing together all the resources currently available in health, education, and welfare in some systematic way. In order for the programs in agencies such as housing and urban development, health, education, and welfare, labor, agriculture, and economic opportunity to be coordinated in an effective way, an agency at the level of the Office of the President—perhaps a Presidential Council of Health Advisers (analogous to the Council of Economic Advisers)—might be necessary. In all of these programs a major emphasis needs to be given to the problems of the poor, since their needs are the greatest. For the medical profession this is not a new role, for one of the fathers of modern medicine, Virchow, in 1848 said: "Physicians are the natural attorneys of the poor and social problems fall to a large extent within their jurisdiction."

William H. Stewart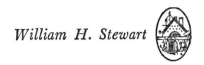

2

Health Assessment

Health is defined by the World Health Organization as the complete well-being of an individual—physical, mental, and social. While this definition is useful as a goal, it is an abstraction and cannot be measured in objective terms. It is not possible to count health. However, it is possible to count death, disability, and disease in a population. Thus, an assessment of the health of Americans is arrived at by examining the burden of disease, injury, and ill-health as reflected in mortality, morbidity, and other statistics, particularly those generated by the National Center for Health Statistics and the National Communicable Disease Center of the Public Health Service.

Definitions

MORTALITY

Deaths are recorded rather well in the United States. Deaths per 1,000 population (the death rate or crude death rate) is the most common measurement of the health status of Americans. The death rate can be examined by cause of death, by age, or by place at death and so on. From these data, disease and injury patterns can be discerned and the distribution of disease and injury by age, sex, and geographic location established. Trends in the death rate over time can be shown, as

WILLIAM H. STEWART, M.D., *who was surgeon general of the United States in 1965–69, is chancellor of the Louisiana State University Medical Center. Dr. Stewart has had a long career in the United States Public Health Service and has written scores of scholarly articles in that and related medical fields.*

well as the effects of new public health measures or therapeutic modalities on death rates.

In studying trends in the death rate for the United States, an age-adjusted rate is frequently used. This is the crude death rate adjusted in order to neutralize the effects of changing age composition of the population, which can obscure trends. The crude death rate will increase for an aging population and decrease for a population that is getting younger even though there is no basic change in mortality. The United States did have an aging population during most of the first half of this century. With the onset of World War II, the fertility pattern changed and the population has grown younger ever since.

MORBIDITY

Morbidity rates—the amount of illness or injury in a population—are more difficult to measure than mortality (death) rates. Morbidity was measured in the United States for a short time during the mid-1930s, but only since 1957 has there been a continuous national morbidity survey by the National Center for Health Statistics of the Public Health Service.

The National Health Survey provides a measure of morbidity in the population due to acute or chronic conditions, including that resulting from injuries. It also provides data on the consequences of the morbid conditions in our society by measurement of the amount of restriction of activity resulting from the illness or injury, such as days in bed or absences from work or school. And finally, it measures some of the impact of this morbidity on our medical care system by recording such events as visits to physicians and hospitalization.

The National Health Survey is our major tool for national measurement of the incidence or prevalence of acute or chronic conditions which result in ill-health of our population. As such, it is essential for any assessment of the health of Americans.

General Disease Patterns as Reflected by Mortality

The United States has experienced a long period of declining death rate. In the first half of this century, the crude death rate dropped from 17.2 per 1,000 population to a level slightly above half that rate by mid-century.

If one looks at a graph of the decline in crude mortality rate over the first half of this century, there do not appear to be any periods where the decline of the death rate was accelerating or decelerating over any other period. However, age-adjusting the crude death rate does reveal two major trend periods in the decline of the death rate since 1900. There was a steady decline from 1900 to 1938 with the exception of the 1918–19 influenza epidemic. From 1938 on, there was an acceleration of the downward trend, most likely the result of the onset of the chemotherapeutic and antibiotic age.

DEATH-RATE TREND CHANGES

The fact that the death rate has declined over the years and is much lower than 50 years ago is generally well known. Much of the existence of medicine and public health is justified on the basis of this decline, and citizens take pride in the growing average life expectancy for their children. Less well known, and extremely important, is the fact that after this long period of decline, the trend of the death rate now appears to have leveled off. In the United States the death rate has been more or less stationary since 1950.

The United States shares this phenomenon of the death rate leveling off with many other nations. From the period 1950–1955 to 1970, many countries have shown a marked slowing down in the rate of decline. In some countries, such as Norway and Denmark, there is even a slight but definite upward trend. And this phenomenon of the slowing down or leveling off is not limited to countries with already low death rates. Even some countries with a relatively high mortality show the same kind of experience.

This failure to experience a decline in mortality rate in the United States since about 1950 is little known, unexpected, and extremely important. It is the implications of this mortality trend that are so important. The leveling off of the decline in death rate, so that the rate has remained about stationary since 1950, has occurred during a period of unprecedented advance in biomedical sciences, development of health services, and money spent to provide these services. The effort put forth in the United States for health and medical services as measured by the proportion of Gross National Product spent for health has increased 20–25 per cent during this period of time (1950 to 1970) during which little change has occurred in mortality rate.

In spite of our concerns about shortages of health manpower, maldistribution of services, lack of accessibility of services, and all the other phenomena gathered together under the heading "crisis in medicine," this country has never had a period in its history when conditions appeared so favorable for health progress. Yet during this time there has been very little influence on our death rate. It is not possible to use overall death rates to evaluate the effects of this enormous effort in health. Other measures will have to be used to justify and evaluate.

SIGNIFICANCE OF STATIONARY DEATH RATE

The demographic significance of the failure of the general death rate to decline will increase over time. For example, a stable death rate means that rate of births is the only variable in population composition and growth. The change in the mortality trend to a stationary rate also has great public health significance. As indicated before, mortality data have long been used as an indication of health and medical progress. If the leveling off of the death rate has resulted from failure to prevent deaths that are preventable, this, of course, is of real significance for the health of Americans. If, on the other hand, the death rate has reached its minimum point, and it is obviously impossible for the death rate to decline indefinitely, this has highly significant demographic meaning over the longer run of time.

CAUSES OF DEATH RATE TREND CHANGES

The recent changes in mortality trends in the United States appear to be based on two factors. The first of these relates to past successes in the prevention of deaths from infectious diseases through chemical and antibiotic therapy. This contributed greatly to the downward trend of the general mortality rate. As the proportion of deaths from infectious diseases decreased, the impetus imparted by the reduction of deaths from these diseases diminished. This leveling off of the death rate from diseases of infectious origin explains part of the deceleration of the rate of decline of the total death rate.

However, a second factor comes into play. The downward trend was checked by the counter thrust of diseases and conditions which constitute the great undertone of mortality in the present population, namely, the chronic diseases and accidents. The direction or rate of change of these trends is such that they would retard the downward course of the total death rate. An example of these diseases is the group of chronic bronchopulmonary diseases which are emerging as a serious public health problem. The death rates for diseases of the respiratory system, excluding influenza and pneumonia, are rising at an accelerated pace. This is particularly true in the older age groups and in males.

Returning now to overall mortality, the decline in the mortality rate and the leveling off of this rate have been somewhat different for men than for women. The mortality rate and the trend of mortality in men do not appear favorable as compared with women. In almost every disease category, the death rate for men is higher than for women.

Moreover, the trend of the mortality rate for women is still downward, whereas the rate for males is decreasing very slowly or not at all.

DEATH RATE LIKELY TO REMAIN STATIONARY

It is difficult to see any major changes in overall mortality in the United States in the foreseeable future, or even much change in the distribution of mortality by age or sex, or changes in the trends within the distribution of deaths by cause during the next decade or two.

Further declines in mortality are possible but likely to be modest. It does not appear that the death rate has reached the irreducible minimum, particularly when compared with the lower death rates already attained in Sweden, Australia, and other countries. But major changes will have to await major breakthroughs in the prevention or cure of the principal chronic diseases. Mortality from these diseases is so weighty that further changes in the mortality from acute diseases will have little or no effect on the overall mortality rate.

Infant Mortality

While the death rate is the most common measurement of the health status of a population, there is universal agreement among public health experts that infant mortality (number of deaths in first year of life per 1,000 live births in that year) is the best and most sensitive index of the level of health of a population, community, or nation. High rates of infant mortality are associated with low socio-economic conditions, poor sanitation, and limited medical facilities and resources. In fact, the infant mortality rate is so revealing as an index of health of a community that given that rate and some indication of the trend of the rate over the past generation, it is possible to describe, fairly accurately, the state of economic development of the community, its age structure if migration is negligible, and the diseases most active as causes of death.

Infant mortality in the United States is lower than it has ever been. Although this is a major accomplishment, the rates appear to have leveled off since about 1950. The rate of decline since that year has been slower than during the first half of the century. As a result, a number of other countries, such as the United Kingdom and Sweden, which had rates higher than the United States in the early part of the twentieth century, today have rates which are lower. Although the infant mortality trend of the United States has been declining somewhat in parallel with other countries, it has been gradually losing ground.

LOW BIRTH WEIGHT SIGNIFICANCE

The specific reason or reasons for the "more rapid slowdown" in the decline in our infant mortality rate are not known. Examination of such factors as age of infant at time of death, cause of death, medical and obstetrical care available, length of stay in hospital at birth, etc., do not reveal any significant differences which could account for the unfavorable position of the United States in respect to several other countries. Of the factors considered, only birth weight is felt to have sufficient effect on the infant mortality rate to suggest it as a possible hypothesis. The effects caused by apparent differences in the incidence of low birth weight infants are of such magnitude as to account possibly for a considerable proportion of the differences between the United States and countries having lower infant mortality rates. Available data suggest that this country has a higher proportion of low birth weight infants to total infants and that this proportion has been slowly increasing.

CAUSES OF INFANT DEATHS

Infant deaths by cause in the United States are largely concentrated in five groups. These account for almost three-fourths of all infant deaths. These five groups include: post-natal asphyxia and atelectasis (collapse of lungs), immaturity, congenital malformations, influenza and pneumonia, and the residual category of diseases of early infancy. There are hidden associations recurring among these categories which are not obvious from the statistics. The thread of prematurity and immaturity runs through a number of these causes, and until we find a solution to premature birth or immature infants, little can be done about the infant mortality rate.

GEOGRAPHIC VARIATIONS IN INFANT MORTALITY

For several decades, geographic variations in infant mortality rates have been recognized in the United States. The highest rates are found in the Southeast. Rates here run about one and one half times that of the lowest part of the country. Urban-rural differentials in infant mortality have been modified since the turn of the century. In the early part of the century, infant mortality was particularly high in American cities. By the time of the late 1920s and 1930s the situation had reversed and children in most urban settings had lower mortality. At present, the situation in a number of major cities is once again reverting to the older position—higher rates in the city than among those infants living elsewhere in the same state.

In the 1950s, there was a general deterioration of and considerable movement into and out from most major cities of the United States. The many elements in the interrelationship of infant mortality among the migrating groups are difficult to unravel because of the lack of quantitative information specific for them. The fact is that pockets of people in areas low in all socioeconomic indicators can be found in our major cities where the infant mortality rate is that which prevailed for the nation as a whole four to five decades ago. Recently, these data have served to pinpoint program efforts by public health officials and the Children's Bureau in this attack on excessive infant mortality.

RACIAL VARIATIONS IN INFANT MORTALITY

About 15 per cent of the live births in the United States are nonwhite—approximately 90 per cent Negroes and 10 per cent other races. Infant mortality differentials have been to the advantage of the white population since data have been available. For the last two decades, the infant mortality rate for nonwhites has been approximately double the rate for whites and, until recently, the leveling off of the nonwhite rate was greater than the rate for white infants and the differential grew larger. The higher mortality among nonwhite infants in the United States is frequently obscured because the trend lines for the combined groups are determined by the trends for white infants since they represent about 85 per cent of births.

LIMITATIONS OF MORTALITY RATE IN HEALTH ASSESSMENT

The infant mortality rate has been an extremely useful and sensitive measure of the health of Americans. By this measure we have never been healthier. But now that the rate is leveling off, it is less and less useful as a measurement of the change in health status of our nation. To be sure, it continues to be useful in pointing out areas of our cities and states where the public's health is 30–50 years behind, particularly among the poor and minority groups. It will continue to be an excellent measure of our efforts to do away with these inequities. And there are indications that the infant mortality rate of the United States will continue to decline and that it will approach the low levels now present in some countries. However, any great decline will have to await more knowledge about and understanding of prematurity and immaturity in newborn infants.

The infant mortality rate, much like the overall mortality rate, will be a much less useful and sensitive index of the health of Americans in the future as the rate becomes stabilized and as we approach a single cause of infant mortality. In fact, neither the overall mortality rate nor the infant mortality rate has served a very useful role since the mid-century mark, but there has been very little recognition of this fact. To measure all the efforts this nation has put forth in health since 1950 solely on its effect on overall mortality or infant mortality gives a completely unsatisfactory answer. Yet this is what we have done for the most part, probably because there is no satisfactory alternative to evaluate the health effort. Other indices will have to be found if the effectiveness of the massive investment in health now put out in the United States is to be measured.

If all that is done now to preserve and restore the health of people within the present state of knowledge has very little promise of further lowering overall mortality or infant mortality substantially, then what is being affected by our efforts and how do we measure it?

General Disease Patterns as Reflected by Morbidity Rates

National morbidity rates are established, for the most part, by the National Health Interview Survey of the National Center for Health Statistics. The National Health Interview Survey is an interview, by trained personnel, every two weeks of a continuous sample of our civilian non-institutionalized population. At the interviews, questions are asked about acute conditions or injuries over the past two weeks or about chronic conditions or impairments present at the time of the interview. If acute or chronic conditions are reported, then it is determined whether or not the condition resulted in a restriction of normal activity and whether or not it resulted in the person's being bed-bound for a period of time. In addition, it is ascertained that the condition reported did or did not result in contact of a physician or in admission to a hospital.

The morbidity rates are usually expressed in three ways: as the number of acute illnesses or injuries over the last two weeks; as the number of chronic conditions reported at the time of the interview; and as the number of days in bed or of restricted activity resulting from the condition. The number of physician visits or the number of hospital admissions is also measured. These latter numbers, of course, give some indication of the impact on the health care system of the morbidity load in the United States.

ACUTE CONDITIONS

An estimated 350–400 million acute illnesses and injuries requiring either medical attention or reduced daily activity occur each year among the non-institutionalized civilian population of the United States. While there is some fluctuation of this rate from year to year, and by sex and age, the fluctuation can be accounted for by changes in rates for upper respiratory illnesses, notably the common cold and influenza-like illnesses. For example, during 1967 the incidence of acute conditions was estimated as 367.5 million injuries and illnesses for the nation's non-institutionalized civilian population. This gives an annual incidence rate of 190.0 conditions for every 100 persons. That is to say every person in the United States, on the average, had just under two episodes of illness or injury over the year, which either required medical attention or resulted in reduced daily activity. Moreover, in 1967 an estimated 53.0 million persons were injured, an incidence rate of 27.4 persons injured per 100 population. Data from later years show a fairly consistent pattern.

CHRONIC CONDITIONS

It is not possible to establish the number of chronic conditions per year as it is with acute conditions. Since in many of the chronic conditions it is impossible to tell when the disease started (for example, arthritis) or since by definition these diseases and illnesses are of very long duration, it is only possible on an interview to get a report of those conditions that existed at the time of the interview, i.e., a prevalence instead of an incidence.

About one-half of our non-institutionalized civilian population reports one or more chronic conditions. In the period July 1966–June 1967, an estimated 96.0 million persons so reported. A year earlier, July 1965–June 1966, 93.7 million persons or 49.1 per cent of the non-institutionalized civilian population had one or more chronic diseases or impairments. In that same survey year, among persons with chronic conditions about 21.4 million people had some degree of limitation of activity. About 6 million had some form of mobility limitation. Heart conditions and arthritis and rheumatism were the leading causes of these limitations of activity and mobility. As would be expected, as age increases, a higher proportion of the population with a chronic condition are limited to some degree in activity and mobility.

DISABILITY

The enormous amount of acute illness and injury in any one year and the burden of the continuing chronic illnesses and impairments result in the disability load in our nation. The extent of this disability burden is a sensitive measure of the health of Americans. It is, of course, a quite different measurement of health than the use of mortality rates for that purpose.

Mortality is an all-or-none phenomenon. You are either dead or not dead. In this sense, it is a static measure of disability or ill-health. When the mortality rate is high, it does serve as a measure of the performance ability of a population. But when the mortality rate is low and it is distributed somewhat evenly among the population, as it now is in the United States, its utility as a measure of the performance ability of a population (health) is limited. On the other hand, disability is not all-or-none by any means. A cause may be disabling in one situation and not in another. A disability rate is much more an index of the performance capabilities of a population, and in that sense, a much better measure of health in a modern society.

Using the year 1967 as an example, there were 1,455,088,000 days of restricted activity during that year in the United States due to acute illnesses or injuries, or about 7.5 days for every person. About two-thirds of this disability is due to two groups of conditions. Respiratory disease accounted for 653,655,000 days of restricted activity, or 3.3 days per person, while injuries accounted for 332,088,000 days, or 1.7 days per person per year.

The number of disability days per person resulting from acute and chronic illnesses, and impairments and injuries, again using 1967 data, was as follows: 15.3 days of restricted activity—5.7 days in bed, 5.4 days lost from work per worker for the currently employed, and 4.4 days lost from school per child aged 6–16 years. In the non-institutionalized population as a whole, about one-half of the days of restricted activity and days in bed are due to acute illnesses or injuries, with chronic conditions and impairments accounting for the other half. Somewhat over half of the days lost from work and about 90 per cent of the days lost from school are due to acute illnesses or injury.

Since not all people are ill or injured during a year, it is possible to examine disability as a person-rate instead of an illness or injury rate. Hence, during calendar year 1967, 22.2 million persons, or 11.5 per cent of the civilian non-institutionalized population, had some degree of activity limitations; this included 8.7 per cent with limitation in their major activity. As expected, the proportion of limited persons increases with age and is higher for males than females in all age groups.

Changing Burden of Acute Diseases and Conditions

The introduction of chemicals and antibiotics into the therapy of acute illness had an accelerating effect on the decline in overall age-adjusted mortality rate. There is little evidence to show that it had any effect on the overall morbidity rate due to acute conditions. However, this may be an artifact since morbidity rates have been systematically measured only since 1957 for the United States. Since the effect of antibiotics on the decline in the mortality rate disappeared about 1950, it is possible that a similar phenomenon occurred to the morbidity rate with the effects of antibiotics on morbidity being lost before 1957. At any rate, there has been no discernible overall change in the morbidity rates from acute conditions in the past decade. However, the advances in immunology against certain viral diseases have been dramatic, and for these diseases there has been a marked change in incidence not reflected in overall figures.

MEASLES

This disease was first thoroughly described by Panum in 1847. Little can be added today to what he said then. Until recently, measles was accepted as a way of life. Everyone had the disease in childhood, usually after he had started to school and then usually in the late winter or early spring. The fact that the disease did kill, albeit at a low rate, and the fact that it left behind brain-damaged children at a somewhat higher rate, were known among medical circles but accepted as consequences of our inadequacy to do anything about it.

All of this has changed with the discovery of a measles vaccine. For the first time in our recorded medical history, it appears possible to get rid of measles. The normal epidemiologic curve for reported measles in the United States usually started from a base line in November of each year, rose steadily to a peak about March or April of the next year, and then fell to the base line by July or August. With the advent of measles vaccine, the epidemiologic curve has flattened out, showing only a barely perceptible rise in the spring. By the mid-1970s, the curve should disappear.

This then is an example of how new knowledge can change the scope and extent of morbidity and mortality in a population even though, as yet, it has not been reflected to any detectable degree in overall mortality and morbidity rates. It illustrates that the changes within the overall mortality and morbidity rates are important when assessing the health of any population.

POLIOMYELITIS

Another disease in which the pattern of morbidity and mortality has been drastically altered in the past few years by research breakthroughs is poliomyelitis. The annual poliomyelitis summary for 1968 begins as follows: "The number of cases of paralytic poliomyelitis reported in the United States in 1968 was 48. . . . In keeping with the pattern which has prevailed in recent years, most 1968 cases were unimmunized infants and preschool children of lower socioeconomic background."

What a change from a decade ago! In 1958, 3,301 cases of paralytic poliomyelitis were reported. In 1959, the number of cases went even higher, to 5,472. But since that peak date, there has been a steady fall in the number of paralytic cases reported each year; by 1970 the few cases reported are the tragic result of scattered breakdowns in our immunization program. This is a dramatic result from scientific effort. Much feared by parents, the season of poliomyelitis was a dreaded one. This has all gone—the fear, the apprehension, the large amount of medical and hospital service needed to diagnose and treat paralytic polio, and, most of all, the three to five thousand children and young adults crippled each year. The health of Americans must have been improved.

Because of excellent surveillance of this specific disease, paralytic poliomyelitis, it was possible to measure the effect of a new vaccine in our population and to say justifiably that the health of Americans improved. Yet, there is no reflection of this effect in the overall morbidity data. The total massive incidence of acute conditions and their disabling effect masks improvements in the health of Americans because of changes in the incidence of one disease.

Poliomyelitis is a good example of how specific surveillance of a disease or condition that can be easily identified is a sensitive measure of any specific efforts aimed at that disease. The conclusion is that any program aimed at the control or eradication of a disease must have a good surveillance effort as part of the program. Only then will it be known whether or not the program did in fact affect the health of Americans.

INFLUENZA

This virus-caused disease is virtually the only remaining disease which still occurs in periodic world-wide epidemics, although not in the severity of the great "flu" epidemic of 1918–19.

The fact that the influenza virus almost constantly undergoes changes in structure has been established. Occasionally the changes are great enough and rapid enough that the virus is almost a new one, and the population of the world is susceptible to the new virus. This susceptibility is so in spite of past infections by a "cousin" of the new virus. Because of this changing character of the virus and the rapidity with which this change occurs, it is difficult to immunize against the disease. The vaccine must be specific for the strain of virus active at that particular moment. Even when this is possible, the protecting power of the vaccine is only moderately good.

In the past decade or so, the world has experienced two major world-wide epidemics of influenza. In both cases, the virus mutation was first detected in the Far East and then spread around the globe in the next three to six months.

Influenza, by itself, is a fairly mild disease but it does lead to complications which can be quite serious, particularly pneumonia. In addition, influenza can activate already existing disease, such as heart disease, and lead to death from that disease.

Hence, in an epidemic of influenza, two other measures of mortality are noted. Deaths due to influenza-pneumonia rise markedly, well over and above the number of deaths expected in that period of time in the absence of influenza. This excess mortality can then be attributed directly to the influenza epidemic. For example, in a recent epidemic, the weekly influenza and pneumonia deaths for Los Angeles County rose from the expected 20–25 deaths per week to a peak of 190 deaths per week. In about six–eight weeks, the weekly deaths were back to the expected normal level. Similar curves can be drawn for deaths from all causes during an influenza epidemic. The excess mortality above that expected for that period of time in normal years is characteristic of an influenza epidemic. The bulk of the excess deaths are recorded as deaths due to heart disease occurring mainly in older individuals.

Influenza is, without a doubt, the major epidemic-occurring acute disease which affects the health of Americans. It has a major measurable effect on the health of Americans. And it will continue to have this effect until research gives a better means of control or eradication.

The specific world-wide surveillance network for influenza is an almost unique example of a mechanism to measure the effect of some new preventive or therapeutic modality on a major disease before the new modality exists. It should be easy to demonstrate the specific and general effect on the health of Americans when it does appear.

ACCIDENTS

Accidents have been among the ten leading causes of death in the United States since the beginning of data collection by state registration areas in 1910. While the mortality rate due to accidents has declined roughly a third over the half century since then, the relative position of the mortality rate due to accidents has risen. In 1969 it was the fourth leading cause of death, a position it has occupied for the last two decades. About 6 per cent of all deaths are now attributable to accidents.

The character of accidents which maim and kill has also changed over this period of time. During the first part of this century, most accidents were at home or at work—and in rural America this was one and the same. Now, of the approximately 100,000 persons to die annually in the United States as a result of an accident, about half are accounted for by the automobile. Home accidents, and to a much lesser extent, industrial accidents, account for the other half.

Deaths from Accidents by Age Groups—As one would suspect, accidents are more likely to rank higher as a cause of death in the younger age groups, chiefly because other causes of death have declined dramatically. In the one to four age group, accidents have emerged as a prominent cause of death, principally because of the decline in deaths from infectious diseases. While the death rate from accidents and violence in this age group has declined, there has been a tendency for the decline to level off in the last few years. Accidents and other violence account for about one-third of all deaths in this age group now.

In school age children, aged 5–14 years, accidents have accounted for the largest proportion of deaths for the past 25 years. However, the death rate from accidental causes has been declining. The rate among white children in 1960 was about one-half of the rate of 30 years ago. The rate of decline for nonwhite children was not nearly so great, but the trend was definitely downward.

The future course of mortality among children five to fourteen years will depend primarily upon death rates for accidental injuries. Accidents account for more than one-half of all deaths among males in this age group. And it was not much lower for females. Because of this, substantial reductions in the total death rate cannot be expected unless greater decreases in the accident rate are obtained. The rate of decline of the present trend of the accident rate is apparently not sufficient to maintain a constant percentage of decline of the general mortality trend.

The pattern of causes of death is fairly similar through the age groups 15 to 34 years of age, with accidents being first or second. When middle age is approached, however, the relative position of accidents falls away as the cardiovascular diseases begin to emerge as the leading cause of death.

Injuries from Accidents—Accidents not only kill but injure and maim many people. It is estimated that about 50 million persons in the civilian non-institutionalized population are injured each year, about one-quarter of the entire population. Many of these injuries are serious enough to restrict the activity of the individual or disabling enough to send him to bed. Accidents by moving motor vehicles, for example, caused about 60 per cent of those injured having to restrict activities and about 40 per cent being put to bed.

The impact of accidental injury on our medical care system is enormous. It is estimated that 10 to 15 per cent of all care in general hospitals is devoted to the accidentally injured.

Accidents in Relation to Health Assessment—It is difficult to assess the health of Americans by examining the deaths and injuries caused by accidents. It is apparent that the relative risk of dying or suffering from accidental injury is increasing in the younger age groups. But this is only because the risk of dying from other causes, particularly infectious diseases, has decreased so greatly. The real risk, i.e., the risk of dying or being seriously injured from an accident when exposed to any specific risk, is much less now than in previous years. For example, the mortality rate from motor vehicle accidents has been falling for some time, if it is measured on an index of risk, such as millions of miles travelled. What is needed are better ways to measure the risk of accidents and the effects of programs on the risk rather than measures of the after-effects of the accident.

The Increasing Burden of Certain Chronic Diseases

The death rate for many diseases of infectious origin, which were once major public health problems, has dropped to a low level. This has resulted in a major shift in the pattern of mortality trends over the years. With the decline in mortality from the infective and parasitic diseases, the relative importance of the chronic diseases as causes of death has increased.

The ten leading causes of death have remained remarkably stationary for the last two decades, with only minor shifts in the rank order. The three leading causes of death—diseases of the heart, cancer, and blood vessel disease that affects the brain—have not changed. These three account for 60–65 per cent of all deaths. In fact, in the list of the ten leading causes of death, only two—accidents, and influenza and pneumonia—would not be included under the category of chronic conditions.

In regard to morbidity with disability from chronic conditions, the same seven condition groups have led all other tabulated causes of activity limitation since the beginning of the National Health Survey in

1957. Heart conditions and arthritis/rheumatism have consistently exceeded all other conditions, accounting for just under one-third of all chronic conditions causing limitation of activity. Moreover, as the severity of the disability increased, they continued to be the most frequent causes of activity limitation, with heart disease exceeding arthritis/rheumatism as the leading cause of disability as severity of the activity limitation increased.

When analyzed as to influence of age or sex on the distribution of most frequent causes of activity limitations, heart disease and arthritis/rheumatism continue to be the two leading causes of males and females over 45 years of age, with heart disease leading arthritis in males and the reverse being true for females.

HEART DISEASE–CARDIOVASCULAR DISEASE

With the overwhelming prominence of heart disease and the larger category, cardiovascular disease, as a cause of mortality, morbidity, and disability in the United States, a special look at these disease categories is in order.

Morbidity reporting for heart disease and cardiovascular disease is grossly understated. Attempts have been made to get a better estimate of the prevalence of heart disease and cardiovascular disease, but they are only estimates. To get some idea of the size of the problem, the following quote from Kerr L. White in his attempt to characterize heart disease in the population is instructive: "In a population of 1,000, 650 have one or more chronic conditions and 400 report them. Included are 150 with heart disease, of whom 60 report it in household surveys and 90 do not."

Comparable figures for all cardiovascular disease cannot be developed; but where data are available, it appears that the rate for all cardiovascular disease is approximately twice as high as that for heart disease.

In the United States there are four major categories of heart disease that make up the bulk of the heart disease group: congenital, rheumatic, coronary, and hypertensive heart disease.

Congenital Heart Disease—There has been little change in the rate of mortality from congenital malformations of the heart over the past several decades. It is estimated that at birth, the frequency of congenital heart disease is about 5 per 1,000. In school age children, early mortality has reduced this to about 2 per 1,000. About 15–20 thousand children are born each year with congenital heart disease. Of these about 35 per cent are detectable at birth. There appears to be little change in the rate of congenital heart disease.

Rheumatic Heart Disease—There has been a steady fall in absolute numbers of deaths each year from acute rheumatic fever and its sequence, including rheumatic heart disease. Indications are that the rate of fall in the death rate from acute rheumatic fever itself has been steeper than that from chronic rheumatic heart disease.

Coronary Heart Disease—But of all the categories of heart disease, the one of greatest concern when discussing the health of Americans is coronary heart disease. The chief concern is the high mortality rate from this disease, particularly in males and particularly in the younger and middle-aged groups. Among white men alone, one-third of all deaths before age 65 are due to coronary heart disease. The rate of increase of mortality from this cause has been particularly steep among the nonwhite population. And the mortality rate continues to increase. While the rates have increased more slowly over the past decade than before, a clear reversal in trend is not in sight.

Hypertensive Heart Disease—Finally, heart disease resulting from high blood pressure makes up a substantial part of the heart disease group. Current statistics indicate that hypertension and hypertensive heart disease account for about five per cent of all deaths and ten per cent of the deaths attributed to cardiovascular disease. During the last two decades, there has been a marked decline in mortality caused by hypertension and hypertensive heart disease. In the entire cardiovascular conglomerate of disease, this is the one which has shown the most dramatic recent change, probably as a result of the introduction of anti-hypertensive drugs.

While the mortality rate from hypertension and hypertensive heart disease has shown the dramatic change to a lower rate recently, it is not known what effect, if any, there has been on primary hypertension in our population. Morbidity data are sketchy and unreliable on this disease. Examination of adults during the health examination survey in the United States revealed definite hypertensive heart disease in 9.5 per cent of American adults and suspected hypertensive heart disease in an additional 4.3 per cent. Hypertensive heart disease is much more common in adult women that adult men and is two and one half times more prevalent in adult nonwhite Americans than adult white Americans.

CANCER

Cancer has consistently been the second leading cause of death in the United States for at least three decades, accounting for approximately 15–16 per cent of all deaths per year. In 1900 cancer accounted for only 3.7 per cent of the deaths occurring in the states that registered deaths. The increasing proportion of deaths due to cancer is a function of several factors: the increase in the proportion of old people; the decrease in mortality from communicable diseases; and a marked rise in the risk of dying from cancer of certain sites.

Sex Difference in Mortality Trends—The trends in cancer mortality vary by age group, sex, and racial group. The sex difference in mortality trends has been most striking. There has been a gradual decline in the mortality rate from cancer for white females over the past four decades and in recent years a slight rise for nonwhite females. However, large increases in mortality rates have occurred for both white and nonwhite males. For each of the adult groups, white male rates increased approximately 25–30 per cent since 1930. For nonwhite males the cancer death rate more than doubled for almost all of the age groups in a similar period of time. This increase among males, both white and nonwhite, and the relative slight decrease in women, is the most remarkable change in the overall trend of the mortality rate from cancer during the past four decades.

This striking divergence in the death rates from cancer by sex is well illustrated by examining the mortality trends over the past 40 years for the age group 55–64 years. In both the white and nonwhite populations, the rate for males in this age group was at a lower level than for females in 1930. However, the death rates for white and nonwhite males have been increasing steadily while the rate for white females has been continuously downward up to the present time. The trend for nonwhite females is slightly upward, but not increasing as fast as the trend for nonwhite males. The trends for the white population crossed about 1945, and those for the nonwhite about 1948. The death rate for cancer for nonwhite males is now much higher than that for white males.

Cancer in Childhood—Cancer has become an increasingly important component of childhood mortality since 1930, when only 0.7 per cent of all deaths under age fifteen were attributed to cancer. Now this entity accounts for somewhat over 3 per cent of the deaths. Part of the rise in proportionate mortality is due to the decline for other causes of death at the same ages, particularly from control of communicable diseases in the intervening period, but it is possible to demonstrate an absolute increase in the cancer mortality rate in childhood. This is due to the fact that the death rate from leukemia has risen rather sharply over this period of time. The two principal types of cancer causing deaths in children under fifteen years were leukemia and cancer of the brain. The sites of cancer dominating cancer mortality in the adult—breast, uterus, stomach, intestine, lung and bronchios—figure hardly at all in infancy and childhood.

Survival Rates—Study of survival rates of cancer patients provides a means of measuring the progress being made in bringing the disease under control. The evaluation of trends in survival is made in terms of the number of five-year survivals or the five-year relative survival rate. The latter is obtained by dividing the survival rate observed in the patient group (crude rate) by the survival rate expected in a group of persons from the general population with the same age and sex distribution as the patient group.

There is no doubt that there has been much improved survival in patients with cancer in certain sites, cervical cancer, for example. For the most part survival rates have improved in those cancers that are slower growing and in those that are located in anatomical sites accessible to surgery and radiation therapy. In addition there has been marked improvement in the length of survival of leukemia victims in response to some of the newer chemical therapeutic agents.

While definite cure is difficult to determine in cancer, it is generally thought that about one-third of all cancers are now cured. This is an improvement from the recent past when it was felt that one in four victims of cancer was cured. There are indications that the survival rates will continue to improve slowly into the future, but any major impact on the prevalence and incidence of cancer still awaits new knowledge. There is little evidence to support any substantial change in the overall cancer rates in the United States population with our present state of knowledge.

CHRONIC PULMONARY DISEASE

Death from cardiovascular disease or cancer account for the vast majority of deaths in our population. From our examination of trends in cardiovascular disease and cancer mortality and morbidity, some gradual improvements can be seen, but major effects on the mortality and morbidity of these two categories await research breakthroughs. There are also indications that other categories of disease are in an upswing and possibly emerging as public health problems. Of particular interest is the trend of the death rate for chronic disease of the respiratory system, excluding influenza and pneumonia.

The mortality from these disease categories has been declining steadily for females, but a sharp upturn may be observed in the rates since 1950. The trend of the death rate for white males was virtually level until 1948 when a large upsurge occurred. The rate for nonwhite males was declining slowly until about 1948 when, as with the death rate for white males, a sharp rise began. Although the magnitude of the rates is still relatively low, the trend for chronic disease of the respiratory system (chronic obstructive lung disease) illustrates an emerging public health problem.

The fact that the magnitude of the rates of mortality are relatively low probably accounts for the recognition only recently of this category of disease as a major problem in the United States. For until recently, chronic respiratory disease, excluding pulmonary tuberculosis, had been one of the most neglected disease categories in modern times. Now lung cancer is recognized as a chronic pulmonary disease that is increasing at an alarming rate, particularly in men. The number of deaths yearly from lung cancer now approximates the number of deaths from automobile accidents.

Chronic bronchitis is now recognized in this century as a major emerging public health problem. Until recently, it was felt by experts that this disease did not exist or existed minimally in the United States. However, it has long been recognized as a serious disease in the United Kingdom and is now one of the principal causes of death in that country. With the advent of diagnostic advances made ten to fifteen years ago, it is now recognized as a major disease in the chronic pulmonary disease category in the United States.

Another disease which is also recognized now as a major health problem is chronic obstructive pulmonary disease, of which emphysema is the most important manifestation. Mortality from emphysema, while rather low in magnitude, has doubled in the last decade.

More important from the health standpoint is the fact that chronic pulmonary disease is quite disabling over long periods of time. The one exception is lung cancer. Chronic pulmonary disease is among the leading causes of bed-days of disability reported in the National Health Survey and is important in terms of disability benefits granted under the Social Security program.

Increasing concern is being generated by the growing number of men disabled by chronic respiratory disease, and by the disruption such illness is causing in the life of the community as well as the individual. This emerging public health problem is of particular significance to the health of Americans since this disease group has been associated with growing environmental contamination in our cities and in certain occupations.

The Burden on the Medical Care System

PHYSICIAN VISITS

The enormous amount of morbidity in our population leads to use of physicians and hospitals to alleviate or cure the morbid conditions. If the health programs were, in fact, making the population healthier, the assumption would be that the need to see physicians or to go to the hospital would decline. In fact, the use of physician services and hospital services is increasing and there is no indication that the trend will not continue. It is recognized that need for health services and effective demand for these services are two different quantities. Effective demand is influenced by such factors as availability of service, ability to pay, and other social factors as well as the underlying morbidity. However, in a fairly well developed country, the use of health services and facilities is an index of the burden of disease and ill-health in that country.

At the present time, there are just over 800 million physician visits in the United States per year, excluding visits to hospitalized patients. About three out of every four persons in the civilian non-institutionalized population see or talk with a physician every year.

HOSPITAL USE

The number of short-stay hospital discharges runs about twelve for every 100 persons. About ten per cent of the population has one or more hospital episodes a year. Most of these people have only one episode in a year, but the more episodes of hospitalization in any one year per person, the longer the stay in the hospital for each episode.

For a long time the trend of rate of admissions to general hospitals has been increasing and continues to do so. For most of this time, the trend line for average length of stay per admission was down. The net effect was that hospital bed-days used per unit of population stayed about the same. Lately, the average length of stay has leveled off and remained more or less stationary. With this change and with the rate of admissions still increasing, the bed-days of use of short-term hospitalization has been climbing.

Thus whatever our efforts to make the health of Americans better, we do not see the effects reflected in the measurements we make of ill-health. Overall mortality rates and morbidity rates, although the latter have been measured only for little more than a decade, have shown little change. In addition, the use of physician services and hospital facilities has increased. Either we are measuring the wrong things and therefore do not reflect the impact of our medical effort on the health of Americans, or that effort, as extensive as it is, is a maintenance effort. It appears that the sum total of what we are now doing in health services is necessary to maintain the health of Americans where it is now. Future effects on our indices of ill-health—mortality rates, morbidity rates, etc.—await major breakthroughs in the state of our knowledge.

Health and Mental Illness

Assessment of the health of Americans by examining the burden of disease, injury, and ill-health as reflected in national mortality and morbidity statistics usually treats mental illness quite separately from physical illness or disease. Therefore, up to this point, all that has been said about mortality rates, morbidity rates, and disability rates has not for the most part included the universe of mental illness. The reason for this separate treatment is not because mental illness is inconsequential. The mentally ill occupy half the hospital beds in the United States. Shortly after every mental health clinic opens, it has a long waiting list. Certainly just by observation, the burden of mental illness is enormous in the United States.

The reason for separate treatment of data on the extent of mental illness in our society is the lack of definition of mental illness which is precise enough to identify a specific illness. This lack of clarity of definition makes it difficult to count cases and therefore impossible to arrive at prevalence or incidence rates.

There have been innumerable attempts to define mental illness and to devise adequate measurement for detection in such a manner that comprehensive mental health statistics could be developed. But at the moment, there is little agreement on definitions, nor is there much agreement on the most appropriate measurements of mental health and illness.

In spite of the difficulty of measuring the amount of mental illness in a population, statistics on mental disorders at both the national and local level are increasingly needed. Despite the inability to use interview survey methodology in the mental field and despite the limitation for estimating total incidence and prevalence of mental disorders from records of patients under the care of mental hospitals or other facilities, these latter data can be effectively used to provide a firm starting point for planning and evaluating programs related to the control and reduction of disability from these disorders.

The first admission rate to a mental hospital system is defined as the annual number of patients admitted for the first time to these hospitals per 100,000 persons in a population exposed to the risk of hospitalization. In the United States, this rate, on an annual basis, runs somewhat above 100/100,000 population. For the last decade, this rate, age-adjusted, has been declining slowly. However, this is not a reflection of a decrease in the amount of mental illness, although modest changes could be masked, but rather is a reflection of the changing pattern of care of the mentally ill. With the extensive development of nursing home care over the past fifteen years, and with the more recent development of community clinics for the treatment of the mentally ill, the use pattern of mental hospitals has moved closer to that of acute hospitals, with higher admission rates but much shorter lengths of stay.

Important changes have been taking place in the diagnostic composition of patients on first admissions. Decreases have occurred in disease of the senium, brain syndromes associated with central nervous system syphilis, the functional psychoses, and mental deficiency. Increases have occurred among disorders associated with alcohol, psychoneuroses, and personality disorders.

The number of patients in the age group 35–44 years has been decreasing rapidly. The number of patients over 45 has also been decreasing but at a somewhat slower rate. On the other hand, in the age group under 15 years and in the age group 15–24, the numbers have increased substantially. This is, in part, an increase in the population in these age groups. But there has been a real increase too. One of the most alarming facts is that while the population aged 15 years or younger has increased by a factor of two, the resident patient rate in mental hospitals has increased by a factor of six, giving a real threefold increase in resident patient rate for children.

As one would suspect, the number of community mental health centers and clinics has been expanding rapidly and the number of patients being cared for in these settings has increased tremendously. In addition, there has been considerable change in the practice of general hospitals in regard to patients with mental illness. Until ten to fifteen years ago, few general hospitals would admit psychiatric patients. Now, admission to the general hospital for psychiatric conditions exceeds admission to the state mental hospitals. The general hospital has become, in many areas, the central axis of the community mental health center.

The measurements cited above tell little about the amount of mental illness in our society. It is difficult, or rather impossible, to say that because of these measurements the mental health of Americans is better or worse. It is possible to say that our modalities of treatment have changed and that the characteristics of mental illness in the various types of facilities have changed. But we have little to demonstrate that our efforts in mental illness, while perhaps meeting better the test of humaneness, are in fact paying off in less mental illness or less disability. We have great need for methods to evaluate what we are doing. Agreement on a reproducible method of defining the mentally ill would be a giant step in that direction.

Dental Disease

Dental disease is frequently overlooked by everybody except dentists when assessing the health of Americans. The rarity of life-threatening dental disease, the lack of visibility of dental disease, both in its manifestations and in the means of correction, and the separateness of the dental profession probably account for this lack of inclusion.

Moreover, it was only recently that national morbidity data on dental disease was available. Previously, data depended on surveys limited geographically and frequently confined to one age group. With the advent of the National Examination Survey of the National Center for Health Statistics, in which a sample of the adult non-institutionalized population was subjected to a modified physical examination including a dental examination, national estimates of dental disease became available for the adult population for the first time. These estimates, considered to be conservative, indicated the great extent of dental disease in the United States. At least one in four adults has no natural teeth remaining in either jaw or both. The adults had an average of 20.4 decayed, missing, and filled teeth per person. About three of every four persons with natural teeth remaining showed some evidence of gingivitis or destructive periodontal disease.

The accumulated effects of dental disease rise abruptly with age. About 1 in every 100 persons 18–24 years of age is edentulous (without teeth). By age 65–74 years, nearly 1 in 2 has lost all his teeth. The mean number of decayed, missing, and filled teeth shows a twofold increase from the youngest to the oldest age groups. The prevalence and severity of periodontal disease in persons with natural teeth also increases with age.

More women than men have lost all their permanent teeth. The number of decayed, missing, and filled teeth is generally higher for women. Substantial differences in dental states were found between white and nonwhite adults. In general, the rates varied by the amount of dental care available to the nonwhite groups. White adults, however, were twice as likely as nonwhite to have lost all their natural teeth either in one or both jaws.

The Health Examination Survey had not by 1970 reported on a survey of a national sample of children. Hence, our knowledge of dental disease in children comes from a multitude of surveys, many as a result of school health programs. That uncorrected dental disease is rampant in children is apparent. The prevalence of disease needing correction far exceeds our capacity to correct it. And, as would be expected, the greatest degree of uncorrected dental disease is found among children from low socioeconomic areas.

It is not possible to establish whether or not dental disease is getting more or less prevalent in the United States since there are few data which lend themselves to trend lines. It is known that drinking fluoridated water will lower the decayed tooth rate in children by 60 per cent. It is also known that the dental manpower available to treat dental disease has fallen behind population growth.

The health of Americans in respect to dental disease cannot be assessed as improving or deteriorating. Until further national data are obtained, only the fact of widespread dental disease can be established.

Summary

An assessment of the health of Americans by examining the burden of disease, injury, and ill-health borne by the population reveals that the national health has never been better in our entire history. The overall mortality rate, the age-adjusted mortality rate, and the infant mortality rate are all at the lowest point in history. Many diseases that formerly ravaged the population no longer exist and others are near extinction.

There has been, however, a most significant change during the past two decades in the trends of the indicators which are used to assess the health of Americans. After a long period of decline in the mortality rate, there has been no significant change in the rate since 1950. The same leveling-off phenomenon is true with the infant mortality rate, although this rate continues to decline slowly. Overall morbidity rates, which have been measured for only about a decade, show little change from year to year. It is apparent that further improvement of the health of Americans, as assessed by mortality and morbidity indicators, can and will take place in the years to come. But these changes will be modest until there is developed knowledge which will permit the large-scale prevention of such a major chronic disease as heart disease or the very common condition of prematurity and immaturity at birth.

The fact that only modest improvements in the health of Americans, as currently measured, can be foreseen raises some interesting questions:

1. What has been done to the health of Americans by the massive investment in medical care over the twenty years from 1950 to 1970, during which time the indicators of mortality and morbidity changed very little? The proportion of gross national product Americans are putting into health has gone up 25 per cent during the time the indicators have remained stationary or only modestly improved.

2. Is it possible that the present effort of this country in medical care, with vast expenditures of funds for this purpose, is mainly to support and to ease the burdens of chronic disease and other noninfectious maladies of man, but has little to do with improving the health of Americans?

3. Are new tools and methodologies needed to assess the health of Americans which go beyond the specificity of measurement now possible with national morbidity and mortality data? Is there a need for data more limited geographically but more specific in its detail?

Answers to these questions and others are required if further progress in the improvement of the health of Americans is to be measured with any certainty. Assuming no major breakthrough in our knowledge of prevention, reliance on the more conventional measurements of mortality, morbidity, and disability will not give this certainty. Of course, the real hope for the future improvement of the health of Americans, for the most part, lies with research and the generation of new knowledge.

Howard P. Rome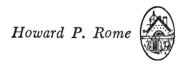

3

Mental Health

Present-day psychiatry is a confluence of trends and issues that is the resultant of many gross and subtle attitudinal changes. These changes have been influenced by philosophical and political elements compounded by demographic shifts in population; they have been swayed by economic influences, implemented and resisted by aligned as well as antithetical professional and sociological forces that are manifest in the psychological sets held by decision-makers and others.

Psychiatry as a medical discipline with a particular social outreach is not exempt from the many shifts and changes that are rocking medicine, among other social institutions. Since it occupies a pivotal position, psychiatry is vulnerable to many contingent spheres of influence that arise within its medical sphere as well as within the sphere of social issues which lie outside the province of traditional medicine. Dr. Fillmore Sanford said this well before the House of Representatives Subcommittee on Health and Sciences: "Mental health is not exclusively a psychiatric problem, or a psychological problem, or a taxpayer's problem, or a legislative problem. It is all of these, and more. It is a problem of the whole social fabric."

HOWARD P. ROME, M.D., has been professor of psychiatry at the Mayo Graduate School of Medicine (University of Minnesota) since 1952. He was chairman of the Mental Health Section of The White House Conference on Health in 1965. President of the American Psychiatric Association in 1965–66, he is now chairman of the Council on Mental Health of the American Medical Association. He has also been a member of numerous governmental panels and task forces. Author of many papers on mental health, Dr. Rome is on the editorial board of five medical publications.

Historical Concepts of Mental Illness

Historically, psychiatry has had the onus of a semantic problem. The definitions and classifications of mental illness have yielded almost as much discussion, polemics, and controversy as the issues of what to do about these conditions. The complexity of human behavior has always been perplexing. Deviant, nonconforming, or bizarre behavior, before and since Homeric times, has been of particular concern to all societies whether primitive or sophisticated. Perhaps the basic puzzle of the precise nature of these conditions is to be attributed to their manifest contradiction of Aristotle's assertion that man is a social animal.

From time immemorial mental illness has had connotations of modes of idiosyncratic behavior that have been labeled by various terms of opprobrium: *lunacy, crazy, bereft, possessed, insane,* etc. The very process of labeling denotes what arbitrarily is held to be antisocial conduct requiring the imposition of social controls. Irony lies in the fact that whereas there is no consensus as to the definition or classification or cause of mental illness, each society has acted as if there were no question about the validity of its assumptions.

There is a not too subtle derogation implicit in the term *mental illness* and its various cognates. These terms cultivate not only disapproval and rejection but a climate of opinion capable of excluding the mentally ill from the moral order altogether. This is just one phase of a subtle process. It begins by locating and isolating a group; then aligning it to the sinful, the deviant, and the destructive; and finally, developing a repertoire of disparaging symbols which depersonalizes the group, thereby completing the stigmatizing process.

Thus, we have first the symbol; then, the accumulation of hostile connotations: unpredictable, dangerous, violent, out-of-control; and finally, the action-issue: the adoption of repressive measures that are institutionalized and legitimized by the rationalization of a need for protection against potential social predators. Thereby we run the gamut of preventive detention in the form of involuntary commitment and indeterminate periods of institutionalization under the authority of restrictive legislation, such as the sexual psychopathy laws and the irony of depersonalization in the name of rehabilitation and treatment.

It is obvious that language in large part predetermines the hypothesis, beliefs, and attitudes that people hold about natural and social phenomenon such as mental illness and health. This confirms Whitehead's opinion that "mankind has consciously entertained all the fundamental ideas which are applicable to its experience [and that] human language, in simple words or phrases, explicitly expresses those ideas." Classification is implicit in language itself by virtue of the logic built into its very words and word-order.

The vicissitudes of the concepts of mental illness and the classifications that have derived from them throughout the past 400 years have swung in a pendulum-like fashion between two poles. At one pole there is Descartes' disembodied Mind and the psychologistic thinking that followed thereafter. At the other pole there is the somatism (the theory that considers all mental diseases to have physical origins) that began with John Locke and burgeoned to an apogee in nineteenth-century positivist philosophy. It is epitomized in Wilhelm Griesinger's slogan: "mental diseases are brain diseases."

For Griesinger and his successors, where brain lesions were not demonstrable, so-called functional disorders of the brain were to be assumed. Ralph Gerard, a neurophysiologist about 100 years later, extended this dictum to metaphorical dimensions by stating that there is no crooked thought without a crooked molecule. Karl Menninger gives a ringing refutation of this as well as a testament to the foibles of all attempts to classify mental disease: "Life is more than permutations in the DNA molecule as the Fifth Symphony is more than vibrating air. And mental illness is more than an aggregate of errors in body physics and chemistry. It is a universal human experience which has a salvage function in maintaining the vital balance."

If the foregoing were only a scholarly debate among different philosophies, it would be of interest perhaps only to historians of science and linguists, but unfortunately, the problem that it represents has implications far beyond mere rhetorical or philosophical exercise. Each connotation has a multiplicity of implications and each implication has an action potential.

The significance of labeling—psychiatric classification specifically —cannot be overestimated. Inasmuch as all operational criteria in every health system ultimately hinge on how many of what variety need what facility in what quantity for their custodial care and medical treatment, the accuracy of the data that are the basis for such judgment is critical.

Extent of Mental Illness and Care

The following data are presented to give some indication of the magnitude of the current problem of the mentally ill. It must be appreciated that the paramount source of these data up to now has been hospital admissions. In recent years, incidental to the establishment under the cooperative aegis of the American Psychiatric Association and the National Institute of Mental Health of a standardized taxonomy of mental disease, reliability of the epidemiological statistics has improved. Annual morbidity statistics on the incidence and prevalence of the mental disorders do not exist for the United States or any other country. The major impediments to their development, as has been mentioned, are the absence of standardized case-finding techniques capable of uniform application from place to place and time to time for detecting persons in the general population with these disorders, and reliable differential diagnostic techniques for assigning each case to a specific diagnostic category, as well as methods for determining the date of onset.

The data presented represent the incidence and prevalence of treated mental disorder rather than the incidence and prevalence of the occurrence of mental disorder.

INSTITUTIONAL CARE

For a long period of time, the state and county mental hospitals were the primary resource for the care and treatment of the mentally ill. In 1946, there were 586,333 beds in 500 state, county and private psychiatric hospitals accounting for 42 per cent of all hospital beds in the country. About 80 per cent of the mental hospital beds were located in the state and county mental hospitals. In addition to these beds, there were only 500 outpatient psychiatric clinics and 109 general hospitals with psychiatric services.

In 1966, beds in state, county and private psychiatric hospitals still accounted for 38 per cent of all hospital beds, and 89 per cent of the mental hospital beds were in state and county hospitals. But, in addition, 1,046 general hospitals routinely admitted psychiatric patients for diagnosis and treatment, another 2,137 general hospitals admitted such patients on an emergency basis only, and 2,148 outpatient psychiatric clinics were in operation. The use of these facilities obviously has changed the nature of the care provided psychiatric patients.

Studies of first admission rates to public hospitals by age, sex, migration factors, marital status and other socioeconomic variables have demonstrated the high toll mental disorders take in every age group; in the lower socioeconomic groups; in nonwhites as compared to whites; in the highly urbanized areas as compared to the more rural; in migrant population groups as compared to the nonmigrant; and in the never-married, separated, divorced and widowed as compared to the married.

Despite the fact that the proportion of first admissions being returned to their communities during the first twelve months following hospitalization increased from 50 per cent in 1946 to about 63 per cent in 1955, the chances of return to the community for those patients not released in the first year diminished rapidly with increasing length of hospitalization.

These patients become part of the hard-core, chronic population and grow old in the hospital. The accumulation of these patients, particularly the schizophrenics, is due not only to the severity of their illness, but also to such factors as: lack of adequate treatment and rehabilitation programs, insufficient staff, depersonalizing effects of a long-term institutionalization per se, administrative problems related to organizational structure and size of hospital, insufficient community resources to help bridge the gap between hospital and community, and a decreased interest in patients on the part of their relatives, friends and the community at large.

Summary studies highlight the increasing rates of admission of patients 65 years and older. Although their duration of stay was relatively short, largely because of the high mortality rates, resulting from their generally poor physical condition at the time of admission, the large number of admissions of aged patients contributed substantially to the growth of the public mental hospital population.

Another factor that contributed to the increase in number of long-term patients was the reduction in mortality in the patient population. This was a direct result of programs that provided better health care for patients and improved their living conditions within the hospital setting. The application of effective techniques derived from public health practice resulted in better levels of environmental sanitation, control of tuberculosis and other infectious disease, as well as improved nutritional status. The application of therapeutic advances in clinical medicine, such as the use of antibiotics, resulted in more effective treatment for pneumonia and other infections. The combination of these efforts resulted in a considerable saving of lives and led to an aging phenomenon for mental hospital patients similar to that for persons in the general population.

The increasing size of the mental hospital population has been a matter of much concern to public health officials, hospital administrators, other professionals, and law makers, as well as the laity. This stimulated action designed to change the situation.

INNOVATIONS IN CARE

During the ten-year period following the passage of the National Mental Health Act in 1946, many innovations were introduced to provide more effective and adequate psychiatric services to the nation as well as additional facilities that were required to meet the rapidly expanding need and demand for such services.

Increasing numbers of outpatient psychiatric clinics were established. Psychiatric services were established in general hospitals at an accelerated rate. Additional nursing homes were opened. These relieved some of the load from mental hospitals, pressed as they were for beds for the aged. New approaches to treatment and rehabilitation appeared: intensive treatment programs were established for the acutely ill; there were total-push programs for the chronically hospitalized; the innovation of group therapy was used to an increasing degree; the open hospital was created which launched various programs for counteracting the dehumanizing effect of long-term institutionalization in the hitherto impersonal environment of the large state institutions.

The introduction of the tranquilizers in the early 1950s was an event of signal importance. It led to greatly expanded possibilities for improved treatment of the mentally ill. The fact that these drugs controlled the agitated and tranquilized the excited provided increased opportunities for using still other treatment and rehabilitation modalities for returning many hospitalized patients to the community. The drugs indirectly helped to develop community programs for preventing hospitalization, as well as for treating and maintaining the mentally ill in communities.

The striking accomplishment of these new agents was the changes engendered in the attitudes of the staff, the patients themselves, and their families. A wave of optimism diffused throughout the communty so that there was a greater acceptance of the notion that treatment for the mentally ill need not necessarily confine them to large insulated and isolated institutions removed physically and psychologically from the community. This innovation reached its culmination in the creation of community-oriented mental health programs.

During the years 1946–54, the numbers of patients in the state and county mental hospitals had increased at an average annual rate of 2.1 per cent. Although the beginning of a change of attitude toward the treatment of the mentally ill resulted in more and more patients being returned to the community, the rates of net release were still not sufficiently high to counterbalance the increasing number of patients still seeking admission. As a consequence, the mental hospital population continued to grow. A major turning point in this upward spiral occurred at the end of 1955, when the patient population reached its all-time peak of 558,922.

CHANGES IN HOSPITAL USE BY AGE GROUP

Between 1955 and 1956, the first drop occurred in the hospital population. This was the year during which the use of tranquilizers became widespread in mental hospitals. This decrease has continued consistently at an increasing rate, so that by the end of the year 1967, the resident population was 426,000, or 24 per cent less than its peak in 1955.

Changes in the number of patients admitted during the year and resident-patient population have not occurred uniformly in every age group. Decreases have occurred in the number of patients 25 years and over, but the annual rate of decrease between 1955 and 1964 varied by age groups as follows: 25–34 years, 2.8 per cent; 35–44 years, 3.3 per cent; 45–54 years, 2.2 per cent; 55–64 years, 0.3 per cent; 65 years and over, 1.1 per cent. Marked increases have occurred in the number of patients under 25 years; the average annual rate of increase for patients under 15 years has been 9.5 per cent, and for those 15–24 years, 5.3 per cent.

The extraordinary rate of increase in the number of patients under fifteen years is due only partly to the increase in the number of children in this age group in the general population. Primarily it is a result of an increasing demand for services for seriously emotionally disturbed children and adolescents and inadequate and insufficient services for them provided by other community resources.

At the other end of the age spectrum, the decrease of numbers of patients in the age group 65 years and over in the state and county mental hospitals has been accompanied by an increase in the numbers of aged mentally ill persons in nursing homes and related facilities for the aged. As of mid-1963, 292,000 persons 65 years and older with mental disorders were resident in either long-stay psychiatric inpatient facilities or in nursing homes, geriatric hospitals, homes for the aged, and related facilities in the United States. This is a rate of 1,662 per 100,000 population 65 years and over. Fifty-one per cent of these patients were in state and county mental hospitals, 5 per cent in Veterans Administration hospitals, 1 per cent in private mental hospitals, and 43 per cent in nursing homes and related facilities. As a result of the increase in the number of nursing home beds throughout the nation since 1963, and the continued decrease in the number of aged mentally ill in state and county mental hospitals, the number of elderly mentally ill citizens in nursing homes probably now exceeds that in mental hospitals.

As a consequence of these changes in age patterns of use, the state and county mental hospitals have shifted their diagnostic composition. Significant decreases have occurred in the number of first admission and resident patients afflicted with senile diseases, brain syndromes associated with central nervous system syphilis, the functional psychoses, and mental deficiency. Increases have occurred in disorders associated with alcohol, psychoneuroses, and personality disorders.

The designation "patient-care episodes" is a statistic which is the sum of the number in the hospital or on the active roles of the outpatient clinics at the beginning of the year and the number admitted to the hospital during the year. This is a count that provides data as to those requiring long-term care. Since one person may be admitted to the same service more than one time per year or to two or more different services per year, this statistic is not equal to the unduplicated number of individuals admitted to services. Special epidemiological studies indicate that of the patients admitted per year to the universe of psychiatric services, consisting of all inpatient and outpatient services in a state, nineteen per cent are admitted to more than one service.

COMPREHENSIVE COMMUNITY MENTAL HEALTH CENTERS

With the enactment by Congress of the Community Mental Health Centers Act of 1963 (PL 88-164), funds were authorized for the construction of comprehensive community mental health centers throughout the nation. In 1965, there were further amendments to this act (PL89-105) authorizing funds to assist in the initial cost of staffing these new centers.

The objective of these programs has been the establishment of a network of comprehensive community mental health centers. These were intended to integrate and coordinate the essential elements of comprehensive service at the local level so as to maintain patients close to their own environment and protect their relationships with their families and the community.

There are five essential elements of such psychiatric service that have to be met in order to have these local centers qualify for federal funds: (1) inpatient services that provide 24-hour care for treatment of acute disorders; (2) outpatient services; (3) partial hospitalization services, such as day care, night care, weekend care; (4) emergency services 24 hours per day which must be available within at least one of the first three services listed above; (5) consultation and education services that are available to the community agencies and professional personnel.

In order to achieve the goal of comprehensive service five additional services are needed: (1) diagnostic services; (2) rehabilitative services, including vocational and educational programs; (3) pre-care and after-care services in the community, including foster home placement, home visiting and half-way houses; (4) in-service training; and (5) research and evaluation.

Nature and Nurture of Mental Health

Of late, there has developed considerable controversy in psychiatry over the validity of what is called the "medical model as an explanation of mental illness." This descriptive abstraction is based on medicine's historical antecedents. Pathology as a construct was used as a frame of reference. Clearly this notion of pathology is based upon the nineteenth-century conception of the germ theory. Clusters of symptoms and signs came to be called "diseases" inasmuch as they were caused by bacteriological agents that invaded the human organism and produced a pattern of function that deviated from normal behavior.

The advent of the germ theory was of revolutionary significance to medicine; its subsequent benefits to mankind have been incalculable. Using this model as a more or less universal explanation, medicine has been persuaded to the belief that all involuntary deviations from the normal, including the emotional as well as the somatic, basically are determined by specific causes, either germs or their homologous equivalents. The point to be stressed is the involuntary nature of the deviation.

Hence, with the advent of the psychoanalytic theory that posited the role of a hypothetical organ, the unconscious, it was assumed that mental and emotional disorders were indeed homologous to the physically demonstrable diseases. It followed that the primary focus of attention was on the individual as the responsible agent for this evidence of what came to be called psychopathology. Then, too, there were institutional derivatives that stemmed from this conception of events. Primary care, treatment and responsibility for persons displaying these signs and symptoms were vested in physicians, significantly called "alienists." Almost by fiat, then, these social deviants were converted to "patients"; by this token they were considered "sick"; and thereupon had conferred on them the dubious privileges of the "sick role." The "asylums" and "retreats" that housed them then became "hospitals." But all this change was in name only—for the most part the stigma and the ignominy which derived from the traditional outcast lot remained. It infused the newly named institutions as well as the caretakers.

The great disproportion between the number of alienists and the persons for whom they were responsible made it necessary to utilize other members of the caretaking team. Until recently there has been no contest of the fact that the physician-psychiatrist, as he is now called, has full responsibility not only legally but also morally, even though of necessity he has to delegate these powers to subprofessional as well as collateral professional groups who are not licensed medical practitioners.

Lester J. Evans points out that medicine is now in the midst of a period of transition and challenge. Secure in its century-old partnership with the natural sciences, it seeks the added collaboration of the behavioral sciences. The most striking phase of this rapprochement is the emergence of health as a value in itself. Disease, most frequently identified by structural change in the body, has been the unrivaled target of medical science; health, conceived as well-being, is now becoming its competitor. Thus, death which was the companion of disease and therefore of necessity medicine's overriding preoccupation, has given way to life. The shift is from dying to living patients, from the signals of danger to concern for something more than the absence of illness as the criterion of health.

COMMUNITY PSYCHIATRY

This shift in emphasis has changed the focus of the search for causative factors of mental illness from those of physical and psychological deviations within the individual to inquiries into the environment in which the individual has literally been immersed. As social scientific techniques became more sophisticated, it became evident, at least in an epidemiological sense, that nurture—learned patterns of behavior —play a vital part in conducing to the development of mental illness. Then, too, this realization gave impetus to the growing dissatisfaction by those who felt subordinated by physicians. They openly challenged the hegemony of medicine as the sole arbiter of the entire field of mental illness and mental health. Shifts from traditional deference to physicians include modifications of the technology and social organization of the delivery of health services. Less and less the doctor stands alone in taking full responsibility for planning and administering treatment of the patient. As the technology of medical care has expanded, so has the physician's dependence upon a team of collaborating health professionals and subprofessionals. The pressure for change is relentless and the question arises, how can the human relations of traditional medicine be incorporated as part of the general preparation of the health services team?

By such progressive increments as these, psychiatry has moved beyond the search for cause within the patient to a focus within the family, and more recently within the environment of society generally. Community psychiatry has as a prominent concern the determination of the demographic characteristics of populations at different risks so as to have the data necessary to plan to meet their needs for special services. The focus of this attention is on the core of social morbidity to complement the traditional concern of the classical model of psychopathology. Psychiatry cannot afford to be comfortable in extrapolating from the personal data it has called pathological to the world at large and its social problems. No longer can it afford the simplistic notion that human behavior and its reactions to psychiatry are the same despite the differential pressures exerted by the several levels of the culture. Psychiatry has become aware of the importance of economics in its relations to social dissolution in a community with its cohort alienation in the individual members of that community.

Generic psychiatry has the role of a messenger contributing to the clinical practice of medicine and its basic bioscience on the one hand and to the burgeoning social sciences and the humanities on the other. It tries its best to orchestrate the intra- and inter-disciplinary cooperation which can offset hitherto parochial views of mental illness.

AVAILABILITY OF PSYCHIATRIC SERVICES

Psychiatrists appear to be located in large numbers where the population is dense, income is high, college graduates are more common and, in general, for the same reasons that other physicians locate themselves in these areas.

An appreciable number of psychiatrists are located in the same states where they had their psychiatric training or their medical training or their college training or were born. The remaining 50 to 75 per cent in any state come from a large number of psychiatric training centers, medical schools, and colleges, so that physical climates and population growth may play a part. The southern and far western states with the exception of California and Colorado have few psychiatrists. Specialists in child psychiatry, mental retardation, and industrial, forensic, public health and community psychiatry are in demonstrably short supply in the nation in certain areas. Practice in social agencies, correctional institutions, general hospitals and mental hospitals is also very low. In short, every area of psychiatric practice is suffering from its inability to meet the demand.

An increase of 23 per cent in the number of psychiatrists while the nation increased in population 18.5 per cent during a recent ten-year period offers some hope, but even this is not enough to meet the demands for many years to come.

The United States pool of psychiatric manpower exceeds 25,000 physicians, according to preliminary studies done by the Division of Manpower Research, American Psychiatric Association. These data include statistics of psychiatric residents. There were 3,969 residents in training at 364 residency training centers as of October 1969; 1,071 psychiatrists were produced by all training centers during the year between October 1968 and October 1969. This survey includes physicians who are members of the American Psychiatric Association as well as nonmembers who have reported a secondary specialty in psychiatry, numbering 4,532.

We are told that we will have 2,000 new community mental health centers by the 1980s. Mental health resources for all of the people has become a goal, not only avowed but institutionalized by multimillion dollar appropriations through national legislation. One needs to know what is the substance of change within the mental health professions generally and psychiatry in particular. Consequently, there is a need to document with specific data the change agents as well as the change they bring about in the institutions of society.

The mentally ill and the services for the mentally ill are no longer provided in what amount to isolated ghettos of a segregated community (the mental hospital). The institutions that house psychiatric practices have been the beneficiaries of political actions that at long last begin to accord them equal rights to health care support.

The time has come when the data of psychiatry can be extended to a scope beyond the headcounts of admissions and discharge and readmission statistics of single hospitals, although these are necessary in order to assess the magnitude of the problem. It is now necessary to have more precise data as a basis for planning. For example, there are five metropolitan states (New York, Pennsylvania, Massachusetts, Illinois and California) which were indicated in a 1965 manpower survey to have within their borders 51 per cent of all of the psychiatrists resident in the United States. When the resurvey was done in 1968, there was a net redistribution of only 1.1 per cent of the total psychiatric population. The far western region led the nation with a 4.2 per cent net growth while the middle western region showed a net loss in psychiatric population amounting to 4.1 per cent.

Child Psychiatry

The development of child psychiatry during the last half century and its well-established position today make desirable that its place and range should be clearly defined in any overview of mental illness and mental health.

Children presenting "nervous" or psychological complaints have been infrequent in the general physician's clientele until lately. Scant notice has been taken of psychological illness in textbooks on diseases of children. One of the reasons for this indifference was that many problems which are now considered as psychiatric were dealt with by educators through pedagogical techniques. Similar to the problem of mental deficiency before being recognized as a discipline requiring medical care and treatment, psychiatric illness was regarded as an educational problem. Its constitutional nature and physical implication were ignored until a later stage of scientific knowledge. There are other factors that have contributed to the recent recognition and expansion of child psychiatry: the beliefs that the origin of the neurotic and psychotic illnesses of adult life are to be found in the experiences of early childhood, and therefore the hope, based on this belief, that psychiatric treatment of children may in fact prevent subsequent psychiatric illness in adulthood.

Then, too, it is assumed that the treatment of mental disorders in their earlier stages in childhood is likely to be quicker and more effective than it would be in its later stages in adulthood. If the mental disorder can be identified in childhood, it is assumed it will often respond to superficial guidance of the child and his family and consequently intensive psychiatric treatment will not be necessary. A large number of children can thus be benefited by a smaller number of mental health workers.

Emotional disorders in childhood are usually based upon faulty personality development, which in turn is probably linked with errors in the child's upbringing by his parents and the community's educational agencies.

The Child Guidance Clinic as a social institution originated in this country in 1917, through the cooperative efforts of the National Committee for Mental Hygiene and the Commonwealth Fund to combat juvenile delinquency. It rapidly expanded its domain of interest. By 1927, it was involved in many avenues of service, each related to preventing or ameliorating adjustment, emotional, and other psychiatric problems in children.

Mental Retardation

A special word must be said about the mentally retarded. Here, too, labeling seems to make a difference. The mentally retarded in institutions are commonly referred to by the generic name "children," but most of them are not children. The word "patient" does not seem a right choice; even though under care, they are not ill. "Inmate" has an undesirable prison connotation. "Retardate" is too formal a designation to catch the popular fancy.

The mentally retarded, like the mentally ill, have suffered more than their share of neglect at the hands of an unconcerned public. It was not until President Kennedy expressed interest in their plight that they were rescued from professional as well as lay oblivion. It was only then that the generic term "idiot" was replaced by the more acceptable term "mental deficient." The institutions where these persons were housed began to be called "hospitals" and "schools" rather than "asylums for idiots and the feeble-minded."

This change was brought about primarily through the indefatigable efforts of parents who were motivated to remedy the social condition of their mentally deficient children. It is only in recent times that the stigma attached to these persons has been diminished and a more tolerant acceptance realized, and commensurate with this, a greater mobilization of community effort in their behalf. Even now, however, there is an attempt by some of their more staunch supporters to stress the need for a clear-cut distinction of the mentally deficient from the mentally ill so as not to have them share gratuitously in whatever stigma is borne by the mentally ill.

Research in this hitherto neglected area of the mentally retarded has revealed the roles played by inherited metabolic and biochemical deficiencies, Rh factor incompatibility, and birth injury. Adverse prenatal conditions, such as German measles contracted during pregnancy and other exogenous factors that cause congenital malformations and premature birth, have been recognized also as etiological factors contributing to the morbidity. Then, too, educational remedial techniques have been made more available generally and have been improved as a consequence of expanded research activity. Further, special classes are being organized in increasing numbers for what is known collectively as "the learning disabilities." No longer are persons with below-average intelligence simply relegated to monolithic institutions; indeed, the institutions themselves are becoming diversified so that they can concentrate special attention on specific kinds of remedial techniques appropriate to the needs of the individual.

However, there is still an unmet need for adequate facilities for handicapped children who do not require institutional care; for those who need special training to remedy their moderate degree of handicap; and for more research into the genetic and consequent metabolic anomalies that are being recognized as the distal factors responsible for these conditions. Primary preventive measures such as these are being incorporated into the expanded nationwide prenatal program in which all pregnant women are urged to enroll.

In October 1963, the Mental Retardation Facilities and Community Mental Health Centers Construction Act (PL 88-164) authorized formula grants to the states for the construction of public and other nonprofit facilities for the mentally retarded. The first grant under this program was awarded in December 1965. Amendments in 1967 extended the program through the fiscal year 1970 and broadened its scope. This was a consequence of an expressed public concern resulting in action at the national level and was the first federal program to provide broad support of construction services for research, community facilities, care, treatment, and training, as well as for university-affiliated facilities providing specialized services for the retarded and clinical training of physicians and other specialized personnel needed in the program.

Between December 1965 and June 1967, a total of 167 projects had been approved for construction of community facilities for the mentally retarded. These will serve nearly 20,000 persons in addition to the 25,000 presently served in existing facilities. The estimated total cost of construction for these 167 projects was 104.1 million dollars, with the federal contribution totaling 30.8 million.

National statistics regarding the problem of mental retardation are extremely limited, and only gross estimates of the number of mentally retarded in the population can be made. On the best judgment of authorities in this field, about one per cent of the civilian population, or two million individuals, require facilities especally designed for serving the mentally retarded. Preliminary analysis indicates that only about 350,000 are presently served in existing facilities.

Alcoholism

It has been estimated, by H. A. Mulford, that approximately 70 per cent of adult Americans drink and that 40 per cent are regular drinkers (drink at least once a month). Alcoholism as well as other complications of problem drinking are a major concern of psychiatry. Seen in broadest scope, alcohol problems range from a basic disagreement about the place of alcohol as a beverage in society to medical complications of excessive drinking, such as the gross mental disorders of delirium tremens (D.T.'s) and other mental disorders due to alcohol.

EXTENT OF PROBLEM DRINKING

The impact of problem drinking is reflected in the large percentage of male patients admitted to state mental hospitals and psychiatric wards of general hospitals, about 22 per cent in 1964, with a diagnosis of alcoholism. This is exclusive of the large number of problem drinkers who receive at least minimal care in the medical and surgical wards of general hospitals. It has been estimated, by W. S. Pearson, that as many as one-fourth of the patients in such wards may be problem drinkers, even though this condition is not usually the immediate cause of their admission.

Problem drinking is found in a sizeable portion of the population; estimates range from 10 per cent to 25 per cent of the families of welfare recipients. For example, in 1965, of the total reported arrests for all offenses in the United States, slightly less than one-third, or 1,535,-000, were for public drunkenness. However, several hundred thousand additional arrests listed in police records as disorderly conduct, disturbing the peace, vagrancy and other charges are commonly known to refer largely, and sometimes almost entirely, to public drunkenness. There were in addition over 250,000 arrests for drunken driving.

ALCOHOL AND HIGHWAY FATALITIES

A clear association has been established between the influence of alcohol and fatal motor vehicle accidents. A recent well-designed study by McCarroll and Haddon established that among drivers responsible for fatal accidents, drinking before driving was three times more frequent than among a comparable group of drinkers not involved in such accidents. Equally striking is the finding that almost half the drivers in fatal accidents had very high blood alcohol concentration—levels over 0.25 per cent, equivalent to ten ounces of whiskey (six to nine drinks)—while none of the nonaccident group had been drinking this heavily.

Figures such as these are only rough estimates. Many of them are known to be inaccurate because of poor records or the failure to maintain any records on the subject. Nonreporting, under-reporting, and misleading reporting are clearly related to widespread community attitudes. These provide a formidable barrier to the rational comprehension and planning of an approach to logical and scientific attack on problem drinking.

ALCOHOLISM AS A MEDICAL PROBLEM

In virtually all American communities, problem drinkers are likely to receive less adequate care than individuals with other kinds of medical and social problems. It has been widely publicized recently, and has been the official stand of the American Medical Association since 1956 and the American Hospital Association since 1957, that alcoholism is an illness—a disease to be treated like all other kinds of diseases. However, the patient suffering from alcohol intoxication is generally not treated with as much sympathy and competence as are most other patients. In the United States substantial barriers persist in the admission of alcoholic patients to general hospitals. Prepaid hospitalization insurance plans do not often include coverage for alcoholic conditions. In most mental hospitals, the level of interest in problem drinking is still very low. As a general rule, few psychiatrists in psychiatric clinics offer treatment for these patients. Public welfare agencies, with few exceptions, have not provided a type of financial assistance for indigent problem drinkers that is usually offered to other needy people.

A particular inhumane instance of the general reaction to problem drinking is the handling of homeless, unattached men found in skid-row sections of all large American cities. They are the victims of the revolving-door system that has prevailed for so many years: arrest for drunkenness, jail for a short period, release to the city streets, and then repetition of the cycle.

Acute alcoholic intoxication can be and often is a medical emergency. As with other acute illness, the merits of each case should be considered at the time of the emergency. Admission of an alcoholic patient to a general hospital should be based on the attending physician's opinion and the behavior and cooperation of the patient. While it is recognized that no general policy can be made for all hospitals, administrators are urged to consider accepting such patients in the light of the newer therapeutic measures and the need for providing facilities for treating these patients.

The major service for the residential treatment of the problem drinker is the state mental hospital. As many as 40 per cent of all men admitted to the mental hospitals in some states are given a diagnosis of alcoholism. Approximately five times as many men as women are admitted to mental hospitals with this diagnosis. Nearly half of such patients are between the ages of 45 and 64 and almost half are admitted on a voluntary rather than on a committed basis. Only about 10 per cent of the state hospitals have special alcoholism wards or programs.

CAUSES OF ALCOHOLISM

The prevalence of alcoholism appears to be markedly affected by social and cultural factors. In underdeveloped countries and among individuals living within a simple culture, drunkenness is generally rare except for periodic orgiastic celebrations in which this, as well as other forms of uninhibited behavior, are permitted in a group setting. In highly developed and affluent societies such as our own, alcoholism is almost universal, but wide variations in prevalence are found.

The age factor is an important one. The graver psychoses associated with alcoholism are shown at a mean age in the late 40s, but they are the result of drinking habits which were begun many years before. Studies show that the average length of drinking history in males before receiving treatment in their 40s was 20–22 years.

A wide variety of physical theories of the cause of alcoholism has been advanced. No evidence has come forward that any specific metabolic, endocrine or allergic factor underlies alcoholic addiction. Although no biochemical differences to date have been demonstrated in humans, there is a good deal of evidence that genetic factors make some contribution to the cause of alcoholism.

It seems plain, however, that social, cultural and psychological factors make an important contribution, and the interaction between alcohol and personality and between personality and social environment must be taken into account in approaching the problem of dependence. Among the social factors that contribute to the initiation and persistence of alcoholic addiction are the approval given in many cultures to the man who can hold his drinks; a substantial consumption of alcohol is regarded as a concomitant of manliness. Alcohol helps to overcome shyness and restraint; it often becomes one of the means adopted by the adolescent to advance toward manhood. Habituation is also encouraged by the conduct of commercial and professional activities over a drink in the bar, or a dinner or social gathering at which a good deal of alcohol is consumed.

TREATMENT OF ALCOHOLISM

Psychotherapy remains the most uniformly endorsed therapeutic approach in alcoholism. Treatment of the problem drinker is nonspecific; some persons obtain relief on a permanent basis, but the major portion of all medical efforts is the control of symptoms.

A community network of services is required to provide the best health care for the alcoholic population. No single health institution or person can hope to provide all the resources necessary to provide for a total population which has alcohol as its problem. There have to be beds available. Community facilities are needed to provide continuing supervision for those who cannot live without some external control. Facilities and therapists for group and individual therapy, half-way homes, day and night hospitals, and training facilities are needed. Counseling service for the patients and their families is required as well as a physician who can regulate the prescribed medication.

A most valuable adjunct to therapy is the organization Alcoholics Anonymous, a loosely organized voluntary association of alcoholics who share experience, strength, and hope with each other in order to solve their common problem and to help others. Dependency needs which are hypertrophied in the typical alcoholic can be gratified through identification with the group or with the new member being cared for, without shame or incitement to rebellion. The active role in helping others serves as a powerful social deterrent to relapse.

The evidence is overwhelming that we cannot as yet isolate a single method or approach to treatment that works for all the affected persons, or one treatment that is clearly superior to others. Many kinds of therapy intervention appear to have been effective with various kinds of problem drinkers. However, the process of matching patient and treatment method is not yet highly developed.

Drug Abuse

One of the unfortunate by-products of the acceleration of social change and the consequent upheaval in our times is the pervasive and widespread use of drugs for non-medicinal purposes. The basic problem is the psychological and emotional state of those who look to the drugs for a solution and thus postpone or avoid more successful approaches toward their resolution. As J. Larner says: "Until an individual can understand his drug need in terms of his own psychopathology, drug use for him will continue to be one of the symptoms that perpetuate its causes."

The drug-use problem is spreading from colleges and high schools to junior high and even grade schools. Certain susceptible individuals, a minority probably representing between 5 and 10 per cent of the population, use sufficiently large quantities, or their tolerance of the quantity they consume is so altered, that drug-taking (including the consumption of alcohol) dominates their existence.

The misuse of mood-changing drugs can be divided into three broad categories: first, the opiates and their derivatives and cocaine; second, the psychodelic hallucinogens, such as LSD and mescaline, plus marijuana; and third, the psychotropic drugs—sedatives, tranquilizers, and stimulants.

In 1965, some 58 million new prescriptions and 108 million refills were written for psychotropic drugs. These 166 million prescriptions accounted for about fourteen per cent of the total prescriptions of all kinds written in the United States in that year. For the years 1963–65, the psychotropic drugs accounted for a steady fourteen per cent of all prescriptions, at a yearly cost rising from 511 million dollars in 1963 to 589 million in 1965. Of every three prescriptions for psychotropic drugs, two are refills compared with the normal 50–50 rate for other drugs.

Evidence of drug use from two current surveys of national samples, one by Hugh J. Parry and one by the Opinion Research Corporation, may be summarized as follows. About one of four U.S. adults uses one or more of psychotropic drugs. Nearly half the U.S. adult population report the use of a psychotropic drug at some time. Stimulants are used by the smallest proportion, sedatives by a larger proportion, and tranquilizers by the largest group. Cumulative use of tranquilizers over a decade has shown a steady increase, from about 7 per cent of the population in 1957 to about 27 per cent in 1967.

There are relatively few significant differences in prevalence of use by major demographic groupings. Major differences appear to be related to sex, religion, and race. Women are markedly higher in use than men. Jews are higher than Protestants or Catholics in overall use and in use of sedatives and tranquilizers, but not in stimulants. A lower proportion of nonwhites than of whites use these drugs; the pattern for both sexes among the nonwhites is fairly similar to that for white men.

Effects of Drug Use

The predominant action of the stimulant group of psychotropics is to enhance and excite psychic functions and to increase motor activity. This group includes the amphetamines and the hallucinogens, lysergic acid diethylamide (LSD), marijuana, etc., whose fundamental action is excitatory. A common property of these stimulants is their capability to induce distortion of perception, hallucinations, and illusions. A frequent consequence of these sensory distortions is the production of delusions, change in mood with its inevitable influence on behavior.

The characteristic of hallucinogens is the perceptual distortion that occurs as an early manifestation in the dose-response curve, whereas much larger doses of cocaine and amphetamine are necessary to induce such psychotic manifestations. Physical dependence does not occur with the use of any of these stimulants so that withdrawal, although commonly associated with fatigue and depression, does not lead to a clearly defined abstinence syndrome. The sedatives and tranquilizers for the most part are substances which reduce mental and physical functioning as their predominant pharmacological action. This same effect follows the use of excessive quantities of alcohol, and is explained as a consequence of a direct action on the central nervous system.

The chronic use of opiates as well as barbiturates is associated with two related but mutually independent physiological phenomena: tolerance and physical dependence. Tolerance is that phenomenon which reduces the effects and consequently requires larger drug concentration to obtain the same effects. Physical dependence is that state of hyperactivity of all responsive tissues which follows the direct withdrawal of the narcotic drugs such as the opium alkaloids and to a lesser extent, alcohol and barbiturates.

Dr. Stanley Yolles, the Director of the National Institute of Mental Health, in his testimony before the Senate Subcommittee on Juvenile Delinquency on March 6, 1968, offered the opinion: "Twenty per cent of the college students have had some experience with marijuana and 5 per cent with LSD. This is in striking contrast to the .5 per cent who used this drug in 1952." What might be termed the experimental use accounts for at least 75 per cent of these statistics. It is felt as a consequence that persons in this category constitute a self-limited problem group. However, even repeated users of marijuana in general have a relatively benign course although intercurrent episodes of mood and behavior disturbance are likely to be more frequent. The use of marijuana is inevitably linked with a proportion of significant abuse, and it is this small percentage of persons that require psychiatric treatment after serious social or psychological decompensations.

A survey by the Food and Drug Administration indicated that in 1962 approximately one million pounds of barbiturate acid derivatives were available in the United States. This one-year inventory was enough to supply approximately 24 one-and-a-half-grain doses to every man, woman and child in the country. An estimated 50 per cent of these drugs were the short and intermediate acting barbiturates, which are particularly subject to abuse.

According to the American Medical Association Committee on Alcoholism and Addiction, there are four types of abusers of barbiturates. The *first* group is composed of persons who seek sedative hypnotic effects in order to deal with their emotional distress. The *second* group contains those persons who have a paradoxical reaction of excitation that occurs after tolerance is developed because of long abuse; the drug now stimulates rather than depresses and is taken consequently to exhilarate and animate the person to so-called increased efficiency. The *third* group consists of persons who take the drug to counteract the aftereffects of various stimulant drugs as the amphetamines; this alternation sets up a mutually reciprocal cyclical pattern of stimulation and sedation. The *fourth* group consists of those who use barbiturates in combination with other types of drugs, mainly alcohol and/or opiates.

Amphetamines deserve special mention. The Food and Drug Administration survey indicated that in 1962, even before the upsurge of drug use and its popularity among the young, over 100 thousand pounds of amphetamines and methamphetamine products were available in the United States. The amount of this one-year inventory was enough to supply 250 mg. of these agents to every man, woman and child in the country—that is 25 to 50 doses per person.

Usually, the person dependent upon amphetamines uses them to cope with such psychogenic complaints as fatigue, failure to concentrate, and a need for a heightened sense of well-being; consequently, he takes these to seek relief from a greater or lesser degree of affective depression.

In June 1966, the House of Delegates of the American Medical Association recognized the serious consequences of indiscriminate use of hallucinogens. In part, their resolution urged strict control and supervision and included the warning that "these drugs can produce uncontrollable violence, overwhelming panic . . . or attempted suicide or homicide, and can result, among the unstable or those with preexisting neurosis or psychosis, in severe illness demanding protracted stays in mental hospitals."

Other hallucinogenic agents have been available for longer periods. Peyote-mescal has been used for the past 150 years by Indians in southwestern United States and Mexico. Psilocybin and dimethyltryptomine (DMT) are relatively new and, therefore, less frequently used.

An LSD "trip," as the perceptual distortion is termed colloquially, is a vivid sensory experience that usually lasts up to twelve hours in contrast to a DMT trip which lasts up to two hours. The subjective reactions and the symptoms and signs are variations on the same theme: distorted perception with varying degrees of mood elevation or depression and a degree of anxiety with commensurate ideational content. Unlike narcotics, barbiturates, and other sedatives and amphetamines and other stimulants, LSD and cannabis (marijuana) have no accepted use in medical practice, with some experimental exceptions.

Neither physical dependence nor tolerance has been demonstrated from the use of psychodelic hallucinogens. Neither has it been adequately and scientifically demonstrated that cannabis causes any lasting mental or physical changes in an otherwise stable person, but this entire question is under study now inasmuch as chronic marijuana users are often lethargic, neglect their personal appearance, and occasionally may experience a deep sense of failure after believing they are capable of accomplishing great things. Then, too, the use of these agents—particularly marijuana—has generated much public discussion and public censure. There are strenuous efforts by law authorities to penalize the users, both those who possess the drug for personal use and especially those who supply it to others. The moral indignation created by the exposure of the frequency of its use by teen-agers has resulted in severe sanctions in every jurisdiction.

As for the psychiatric picture, the signs and symptoms of marijuana intoxication are primarily subjective. The user experiences some of the following effects: a feeling of well-being, hilarity, euphoria, distortion of time and space perception, impaired judgment and memory, irritability and confusion. There is frequently a hypermobility without impairment of coordination. It is significant that the environment influences to a large extent the quality and quantity of a user's reaction. Then, too, the kind of a person he is—his habitual style of response—has a bearing upon the response of the user. When burned, the smoke of pot has a characteristic acrid odor so that there is little difficulty in recognizing the intoxication of a person who has smoked a significant amount of marijuana in the preceding few hours.

Criminal Responsibility of the Mentally Ill

The thorny issue of criminal responsibility for acts committed by the mentally ill has been a source of concern and controversy since the decision of the judges in the M'Naghten case in England in 1843. That year saw the advent of the "right and wrong" test incidental to which fifteen judges were summoned before the House of Lords to express their opinions about an unpopular verdict in which M'Naghten, who had killed the Secretary of the Prime Minister, Sir Robert Peel, was acquitted on the ground of insanity. The judges made the statement that the "party accused was laboring under a defective reason, from disease of the mind, as to not know the nature and quality of the act he was doing, or if he did know that he did not know he was doing what was wrong."

With the exception of the modification of the ancient doctrine of *mens rea* (guilty mind) by the concept of an "irresistible impulse" in 1887, it was not until 1954 that there was another test promulgated to supersede the knowledge of right and wrong test of the M'Naghten rule. The Durham decision, which is the governing rule in the District of Columbia, states that "an accused is not criminally responsible if his unlawful act was the product of mental disease or mental defect." Under this test, culpability is determined not on the basis of some hypothetical state of mind of the defendant, but by a judgment as to whether the offense derived from the mental illness of the defendant.

Subsequent to the Durham decision, there has been a considerable elaboration of this rule by decisions which in effect change the notion of criminal behavior as being the "product" of mental disease. The more acceptable test, in the wording of the Currens decision handed down in 1961, is: "lacked substantial capacity to conform."

In this area, again, one hears *pro* and *con* discussions based on semantic connotations—another form of the labeling question which has plagued psychiatry from its beginnings. Here, too, the substantive issues are beclouded by one's politico-philosophical leanings: in the parlance of the present day, whether one is a strict constructionist (conservative in this viewpoint) or inclined to a more liberal approach. In the latter case one stretches laws and rules to better fit people found guilty of infractions. In the former case one adheres closely to the rule of law motivated by the conviction that social order depends on blind justice which is even-handed and impartial. Proliferations of this controversy have far-reaching effects. To illustrate, there is the as-yet-unresolved problem of the so-called sexual psychopath and the issue of preventive detention that in some instances amounts to a life sentence.

Then, too, the dilemma of involuntary commitment and the legal issues raised about its infringement on human rights is actually a conflict between the civil rights and liberties of the individual on the one hand and the rights of society on the other. It appears that in most cases, under our present statutes, a person is in actuality committed because (1) he is talking or acting in a way that seems peculiar to his family or the community, and (2) the family and/or community considers this behavior threatening or unacceptable and will not tolerate it within its own setting.

These times of protest and dissent, often threatening, lend currency to the long-neglected problem of the abrogation of the civil rights by involuntary commitment of those said to be mentally ill.

Summary

A comprehensive overview of mental illness and mental health is necessarily a difficult task. There are numerous variables whose influences must be taken into consideration. The validity of the basic assumptions upon which they rely also have to be taken into account, for they are influenced by the personal beliefs and attitudes of the viewer as well as those whose activities are being judged. In the over-all, it can be said that the progress in psychiatry and its allied fields, particularly since World War II, has been great. In part, this has been through the efforts of citizen groups that have mobilized a generous public response and endorsed in large measure the programs recommended by the professionals.

This progress has taken many forms. The traditional place for the treatment of the mentally ill has been moved from its almost total commitment within institutions to outpatient facilities located in the community independent of and in connection with other health-caring activities. Moreover, there has been an acceptance by the community of the "new way" of providing care.

The status of current mental health concepts, which in part have been responsible for the intent and direction of these activities, is diffuse. In the first place, mental health is a broad term and its activities are legion, involving the functions of the individual, masses of the population, and professionals in many disciplines. Its task has involved a multiplicity of systems of thought and range of methods of attack as heterogeneous as the individuals, groups, and disciplines involved in the problem. Mental health activities, therefore, often have a flavor of morals and ethics, religious fervor, personal investment, unvalidated psychological concepts, value judgments, psychiatric theory, political science, welfare movements, and cultism. In other words, when one considers the broad area of mental health and the preventive measures which its attainment implies, he is immediately involved in social issues which lie outside of what customarily is thought to be the proper province of medicine.

In partial recognition of this, the citizen's movement in this area has not been constrained narrowly within the province of defined mental illness, but rather has ranged broadly to such related fields as education on the one hand and remedial measures to offset the devastating effects of poverty on the other. Thus, certain trends and basic assumptions have served as focal points for the concentrated efforts of the National Institute of Mental Health in addition to what would customarily be thought of as the proper province of a federal health activity.

As Marie Jahoda points out:

> Perhaps the greatest handicap for a systematic study of the social conditions conducive to mental health is the very elusiveness of this concept. As far as we could discover, there exists no psychologically meaningful and, from the point of view of research, operational description of what is commonly considered to constitute mental health.

Thus, one arrives at multiple criteria for determining the mental health of an individual and considers such things as an active adjustment or attempts at mastery of his environment as distinct both from his inability to adjust and from his indiscriminate adjustment through passive acceptance of environmental conditions. Then, too, there is the unity of his personality, the maintenance of a stable, internal integration which remains intact notwithstanding the flexibilty of behavior which derives from active adjustment. And finally, there is the ability to perceive correctly the world and himself.

The term *mental health* is said to emerge from public health practice and to constitute the generic problem of psychiatric disorders in large populations. The term *mental hygiene* carries the connotation of prevention although it too is not specific. The word *mental* refers commonly to cognitive functions, and the word *health* is used often when disease is under consideration. As a concept then, mental health is comprised of multidimensional referents and suggests inferences to multiple areas of human behavior and pathology.

Inasmuch as the emphasis in mental illness has shifted to include exploration of the field of prevention, with many and varied programs geared in that direction, the thrust of this exploration has been at removing the causes of such illness. This effort has moved in the direction of the social sciences and their application to psychiatry, in terms of the environmental setting in which presumed etiological factors become enhanced.

Considered as primary is prevention, a modification of life conditions in such a way that disorder does not ensue. Considered as secondary is prompt and effective treatment, which prevents the development of more serious symptoms and complications and/or the reduction of symptoms to a lesser degree of intensity.

It goes without saying that a program for scientific prevention must ultimately be based on an adequate knowledge of etiology, modes of transmission, and techniques for the eradication of causative as well as precipitating agents. Definite causes of mental and emotional diseases are essentially unproved by these scientific criteria. Consequently, mental health as a scientific concept is essentially still in the stage of hypothesis making and testing.

Suffice it to say that mental and emotional illnesses, with few exceptions, are not "due" to any one or a number of things in a strict etiological sense, but represent patterns of reaction, in a given social and cultural environment, to the myriad of factors which influence the individual.

The observation of Alfred North Whitehead is fitting: "A civilization which cannot burst through its current abstractions is doomed to sterility after a very limited period of progress."

William N. Hubbard, Jr.

4

Health Knowledge

The idea of health itself is a human value judgment. The term is ideally defined as well-being, in physical, mental and social realms. In the most common usage, however, health refers to an absence of a specific disease or disability. Health is an enabling value rather than a definitive purpose. To achieve it is to be in the condition that allows fulfillment of one's potential. Health pursued for its own sake is a fetish. Because it functions by enabling other purposes, health must also be recognized as having a relative rather than an absolute value, one of the many factors that are together essential to an ecologic balance favoring mankind.

An essential element of human health is the survival of the species; but a more satisfying concept is a state free of impediment to the fulfillment of human potential. Within these limits there are two continuing forces whose resultant vector provides the dynamic and continually evolving human condition. The first of these, the biological evolution of man, has been relatively successful in terms of man's domination over other competing species and his adaptation to and control of his terrestrial physical environment. His health will con-

WILLIAM N. HUBBARD, M.D., *is vice-president and general manager of the Pharmaceutical Division of The Upjohn Company. Until recently he was dean of the Medical School of The University of Michigan. He is a member of the Board of Directors of the National Board of Medical Examiners and of the Governor's Advisory Commission on Education for Health Care. Dr. Hubbard was chairman of the Board of Regents of the National Library of Medicine in 1965–67 and president of the Association of American Medical Colleges in 1967–68.*

tinue to be dependent on this biological evolutionary success. For the past 50,000 years, the cultural pressures exerted by man's living in ever larger and more complex groups have become the second and most troublesome force determining the human condition.

Man's survival is now threatened by the results of the interaction of his more recent cultural evolution and his underlying biological evolution. The limitations on the fulfillment of human potential are now predominantly of cultural origin. It is to be emphasized, however, that a separation of the biological and cultural forces is useful only for the purposes of analytical description. In fact, these two forces are inseparable, interacting components that modify each other to form the changing definition of man.

From the point of view of the biologist, the idea of human health is difficult to treat scientifically. Reproductive fitness and the capacity of the species to adapt to environmental stresses while surviving over extended generations is a scientific statement of biological success that is analogous to health. Genetic information accumulated over millions of years of biological evolution and changing slowly in response to environmental pressures, both physical and cultural, is the elemental biological definition of the human species. Whatever contributes, therefore, to reproductive fitness and species survival would be interpreted in strict biological terms as health.

For several thousand years religious, political, and humanistic values have contributed important cultural elements to the elementary biological definition of health. The sanctity and significance given the individual human being have varied with the economic success and political form of our social structures. Fostering longevity beyond the point where independence and productive effort are maintained is now a generally accepted social goal. Supporting the survival, if not the reproduction, of individuals who have physical or mental limitations at birth that make independence or productivity highly improbable is likewise a current social goal. The extent of the resources that are made readily available by society to sustain and restore the health of individuals threatened by disease or accident has become a generally accepted measure of the validity of sociopolitical structures. Indeed, these social goals have become so prominent today that they have begun to consume a distressingly large share of the gross national product of the United States. These social goals related to health tend to be stated in absolute terms. There is no natural limit placed on the allocation of resources to support direct health services with the single exception of the competition with competing demands from other essential social services. One of the most compelling problems facing the United States today is to develop a logic by which the relative benefit of resources devoted to the support of personal health services can be determined in comparison with the benefit of equivalent resources being devoted to other essential functions of the society.

Science and Health

Rene Dubos has suggested that scientists might find it useful now and then to evaluate their professional activities in the light of Kant's admonition:

> To yield to every whim of curiosity, and to allow our passion for inquiry to be restrained by nothing but the limits of our ability, this shows an eagerness of mind not unbecoming to scholarship. But it is wisdom that has the merit of selecting from among the innumerable problems which present themselves, those whose solution is important to mankind. (Emanuel Kant, 1766, *Dreams of a Ghost Seer,* 3rd chapter.)

Until the twentieth century, biomedical research was characterized by a direct concern with disorders that resulted in premature death. Until the middle of the nineteenth century, medical and health-related knowledge were accumulated almost entirely through the empirical approach of trial and error experience. The inherent authoritarianism of such empirical knowledge made its usefulness erratic, but its achievements in controlling disease were nevertheless impressive. Even in the latter half of the nineteenth century, however, quinine was the only specific curative agent available and the infectious diseases remained, as they had been throughout man's entire history, the great wasters of human life. As biology adopted the experimental methods of the physical sciences, a powerful new strategy became available to the biomedical investigator. During the latter half of the nineteenth century both psychiatry and psychology independently moved also toward objective and even quantitative analytical systems. Specific problems of human health were attacked by this new experimental scientific strategy.

EXPERIMENTAL RESEARCH EFFORT

The new experimental research effort was initially fostered by the German universities and later by governmentally supported institutes in both France and Germany. In the United States it was the great private philanthropic foundations working both through the universities and through their own institutes that began to bring the advantages of intensive biomedical experimental research to the United

States in the early part of the twentieth century. Shortly thereafter the federal, city and state health departments began to support intramural and some extramural research.

It was not, however, until World War II that massive tax support of biomedical research was initiated. Facing problems of traumatic shock, malarial infestation, epidemic typhus, wound infection and a host of other specific health problems, highly organized efforts were instituted to apply experimental scientific research to discovering the knowledge necessary to solve the problems. Fundamental research, applied research and the technology of distribution of services to the place of need were joined together with a spirit of submission of self-interest to public purpose. The result of this programmed effort was a series of brilliant achievements. Antibiotic and chemotherapeutic agents effective against a long list of diseases were developed. Blood fractions and blood substitutes were developed along with methods of blood storage which allowed surgical repair of trauma that had historically been fatal. The utility of scientific biological knowledge in solving problems of human health was demonstrated with impressive emphasis.

Within five years after the conclusion of World War II there began an extraordinary growth of support of research in the biological sciences that are basic to medicine as well as in the clinical sciences themselves. Between 1948 and 1968 the total national support annually for medical research rose from an estimated $124 million to $2.5 billion. During this interval the National Institutes of Health increased their annual expenditures from approximately $20 million to almost $1 billion.

NATIONAL PRIORITY SHIFT FROM RESEARCH EFFORT

By 1965, the funds from the National Institutes of Health assigned to extramural research in the universities of the United States had ceased to increase and in the succeeding years, measured by a level dollar value that accounted for inflationary changes, the level of research support decreased significantly. Beginning in 1965, however, there was a sharp increase in the total federal expenditures for personal health services. Although these changes were not immediately apparent to the general public, by 1970 it became obvious to even the most casual observer that federal priorities had sharply shifted from the support of research to the support of direct personal health services.

The question was increasingly asked during this five-year interval as to whether the shifting priority was killing the goose that laid the golden eggs or whether the research establishment since the middle fifties had itself laid an egg. After the middle fifties the life expectancy of people in the United States did not continue the increases that had begun 30 years before. Specific prevention of cancer and heart disease had not flowed from massive research into these problems. Therapy for cancer and heart disease could hardly be described as reliably curative. Most troublesome of all was the lack of a convincing explanation of the probable relationship between the intellectual interests of the biomedical researcher and the solution of the most urgent health problems perceived by the people of the country. After almost 30 years of unquestioned support of basic and applied biologic and medical research, in the last half of the 1960s the growth of this support stopped and a national debate grew as to whether there was a continuing relationship between improved scientific knowledge and improved health.

Quite erroneously there was support at the highest levels for the notion that a large amount of knowledge that had direct applicability to improving health was somehow sequestered in laboratories or research institutions and not made available to the general public. The fact of the matter is that the obvious deficiency noted in delivery of health services according to need was not significantly related to the movement of the best knowledge and practices into the technology of those services. Rather, the real impediments were the inadequate volume of services produced and the limited capacity to distribute them universally according to need. Unfortunately, the idea grew and was fostered by well-intentioned and misguided spokesmen for the national interest that in effect we had done enough for research for a while and should now busy ourselves with applying this research-derived knowledge to the practical solution of our health problems. The superficial plausibility of this erroneous advice greatly supported both the legislative and the executive branches of government in their decision to reduce the support of research. The tragedy of this judgment is that continuing growth of research is essential. The optimum distribution of our present level of knowledge—or more exactly of our ignorance—will not resolve the most pressing health problems of our time. Dollars saved by reducing research expenditures are orders of magnitude smaller than the dollars necessary to support the personnel and facilities required to produce and distribute our best health services to everyone in the United States who needs it.

The more fundamental question is whether the particular strategy of biological research for the last 25 years has a high probability of producing knowledge relevant to the solution of urgent health problems. An even more troublesome question is whether the fields of inquiry encompassed by biology and the biological aspects of clinical medicine are themselves the fields that are relevant to the most pressing problems which limit man's health and threaten his actual survival.

Urgent Health Problems

POVERTY

Poverty-specific death and disease rates are the most immediate problems of health in the United States. Where specific curative measures for acute disease exist, they are usually available even though awkwardly to rich and poor alike. On the other hand, where the disabling effects of disease can be prevented by early detection and prompt therapy or can be limited by long-term supportive care, there is a disastrous difference in the availability of personal health services to the rich and to the poor. The most flagrant example of this is in the infant death rates, which vary in almost exact inverse relationship to the economic status of the individual. The appearance of psychiatric disorders and the disabling effects of chronic disease follow this same appalling pattern. It is of high significance to understand that these discrepancies between the health of the rich and the poor are not based on defects of scientific knowledge but rather are defects in the production and the distribution of health services.

OVERPOPULATION

The long-range problem most seriously threatening America's health is the excessive rate of growth of our population. Although crude birth rates have declined since World War II and before that had been declining for approximately 50 years, the growth of the population is now excessive. This occurs because the number of people in the child-bearing age has grown at a rate much greater than the decrease in the rate of births per individual. Adding to this is the extended life expectancy which retains each person born as part of the total population for almost 30 years longer than at the beginning of the century. The percentage of our population in the economically non-productive younger and older age brackets continues to increase.

It would be amusing, if it were not so threatening, to contemplate a federal agency preparing to ban contraceptive agents that have any demonstrable risk to the patient even when these risks are statistically less threatening than the pregnancy that is being prevented—much less the assured deleterious burden of an unwanted child. This same macabre sense of humor can be satisfied by considering abortion laws which deprive a woman of the right to decide whether or not she will bear a child; by noting that income tax laws are written to give advantage that increases directly with the total number of children in the family; and, finally, by watching child abuse and child abandonment increase at tragic cost to the development of the child and at great expense to the public while legislative arguments continue on the assumption that there is public benefit in an unwanted pregnancy.

THE AGED

The support of older people who are economically and personally no longer independent is a health problem of explosive growth potential. The principal cause of this age-related disability is generalized occlusive arteriosclerotic disease of the heart, brain, and extremities. Associated so-called degenerative diseases such as osteoarthritis, diminished auditory and visual acuity, emphysema, and late onset diabetes contribute heavily to disability in the aged. None of these age-related disorders can be reliably prevented and none has specific cures. All are compatible with many years of life, the extent varying with the degree of supportive care. This problem is so formidable that it is characteristically excluded from private and public discussions of provision of personal health services. The aged do not have specific disease episodes that lend themselves to neat actuarial prediction. Their care does not demand "skilled nursing" services on a daily basis. There is no conclusive end point to their treatment. Most are not completely dependent, either economically or physically, but few are self-sufficient. The knowledge and experience to deal with this health problem do not exist.

DESTRUCTIVE BEHAVIOR

The goddess Hygeia was the classic patron of health and the idea of hygiene is properly derived from her. Because man is self-aware and within some statistical limits self-determining, his choice of action will heavily influence his state of health. Genetic heritage, cultural conditioning, life experience, and the quality of the environment all limit an infinite sort of self-determination. Some destructive behavior has been classed as "disease" on the assumption that it is not self-determined but caused by forces "outside the control" of the individual. The implication is that the individual is "blameless." The counter-argument is that "no one forces" the behavior and therefore the individual is "responsible" or "gets what he deserves."

An enormous amount of human energy has been wasted on this feckless argument that has at its root the legalistic adversary strategy for assigning blame. The futility is that even if blame for an occurrence of destructive behavior could be accurately assigned and punished, the causes of the behavior would not have been effectively altered. Our knowledge and skill in dealing with this set of problems are so rudimentary that we are unable even to collect valid empirical information about the phenomena. Together these phenomena are now the greatest wasters of productive years of life in America.

ACCIDENTS

Accidents are the greatest cause of death in the younger age group and therefore the greatest single waster of years of productive life. The greatest single cause of fatal accidents is automobile collisions. Most of the fatal accidents are related to the abuse of alcohol and are also highly related to prior aggressive behavior patterns in the driver who is involved in a fatal accident. Although highway accidents are a matter of real concern, the majority of fatal accidents occur at speeds below 40 miles per hour within twenty miles of the driver's home.

OBESITY

It has been reliably estimated that if obese individuals were reduced to ideal weight, the average life expectancy in the United States would increase by seven years or more. The significance of this is illuminated when one calculates that if all forms of cancer were to be removed, the average life expectancy of the people of the United States would increase by only two to three years. It is also assuredly true that there are many more years of life in the United States wasted because of obesity than are wasted because of under-nutrition.

INDOLENCE AND SMOKING

If physical indolence and smoking along with obesity are observed in relationship to the occurrence of death and disability from coronary heart disease, it becomes painfully evident that even though they may not determine the occurrence of occlusive atherosclerotic coronary vascular disease itself, they are of very high importance, indeed, in determining whether such disease causes death or disability. Pulmonary emphysema is the most rapidly increasing age-related disabling disease in the United States. Although obstructive emphysema has complex origins, its incidence has a direct relationship to the frequency and amount of cigarette smoking. The much less common but more dramatically revealed deaths from cancer of the lung have a similar statistical and probably causal relationship to cigarette smoking.

Physical indolence erodes stamina, predilects to insomnia, statistically correlates with hypertension and obesity and, as well, commonly coincides with psychic depression. The sedentary musculo-skeletal and the highly stressful psychologic pattern of urban life is a combination for which there are no adaptive mechanisms from biological evolution. Our knowledge of the so-called diseases of stress arising from this biologically paradoxical life style is minimal, but tentative observations confirm that hypertension, peptic ulcer, anxiety neuroses and strokes as well as deaths from coronary artery disease are of highest frequency in the urban setting. This realm of health-related knowledge is still predominantly intuitive in character.

ALCHOLISM AND DRUG ABUSE

Alcoholism and other forms of drug abuse are second only to the major psychoses as a cause of morbidity in the 20–60 year age group. Drug abuse and defective mental health are so closely interrelated that it may not be possible to discuss them separately. On the other hand, alcoholism and drug abuse commonly occur in the absence of specific psychiatric disorders while the converse is equally true.

Alcoholism, drug abuse and so-called psychoneurotic behavior are clearly inimicable to human well-being. On the other hand, they do not fit the traditional usage of the term "disease" since they have a significant component of self-determined choice in their origins. Because of this element of self-determination, there is a strong bias in our culture toward assigning blame to the individual and a reluctance as well to deal with the complex set of fundamental causal factors.

This group of health-limiting conditions displays most starkly the interdependence of cultural and biological forces in establishing the human condition. The presently applied logic of scientific explanation and our existing research strategy to define causal relations cannot deal with the degree of complexity that these phenomena contain. The multiplicity of variables that act interdependently with an orderly rather than random simultaneity represents a single system that is now largely a "black box." Even to describe, much less manipulate, this bio-social system requires an ecologic approach that is presently in the earliest stages of conceptual development. Only from such a matured ecologic strategy will knowledge necessary for remedial action come.

Biomedical Research as a Problem

Consider the foregoing list of threats to man's health and survival: inadeqaute production and distribution of personal health services, excessive population, obesity, accidents, alcoholism and drug abuse, smoking, physical indolence and, to complete the roster, suicides—the largest cause of death among college students. These disorders have their determinants in cultural, economic and social factors which fall far outside the central intellectual interests of modern biological research. It is not even clear that these are disorders that fall within the ordinary definitions of disease. Certainly they are not the kind of problems that will have a single specific therapeutic agent or a specific medical treatment. The approach to their management must be ecologic rather than through pursuing a description of these phenomena at the molecular level.

More important for this discussion of the relationship of knowledge to health, the control of these impediments is a problem not only of the absence of knowledge but also of the utilization of existing and future knowledge through education, laws, and adequate health services. The impediments to utilization are political, economic, cultural, and sometimes religious. A major education effort is necessary to provide the intellectual and social base of the changes in behavior required to deal with these health problems. When one begins to suggest increased taxation; to threaten the continuing existence of the cigarette manufacturers; to criticize the industries that build our automobiles and maintain our highways; to invade the rights of the food industry to urge high caloric fatty preparations on an over-fed and sedentary population; and to threaten the right of individual citizens to operate a vehicle or to accept responsible employment when habitually under the influence of alcohol or drugs, we then enter into the true dilemma of improving health. This real dilemma is the contest between the value assigned to health and the value assigned to competing activities that may be antagonistic to health.

Securing the health of Americans is a goal that goes far beyond the traditional provision of health services by physicians, dentists, nurses and related workers. Both political and economic stability are prerequisites to health of the population. General education and specific health-related education, especially for parents and teachers, are essential to the fostering of those determinants of health that are personally controlled by the individual. The consumption of essential nutrients in an amount that does not grossly depart from the minimal requirements of the individual requires a highly informed balance between availability and personal restraint. The goal of true sanitation of the environment is frequently beyond the reach of the individual's efforts and is in a spectacular contest with the competing goal of maximum economic advantage in the use of environmental resources. Both public and personal health care require a rational and coherent system for their delivery to the point of need in the face of economic, cultural, and geographic barriers. If knowledge related to health is to be effective in contributing to well-being, then these barriers to health must be recognized and systematically surmounted through informed political action.

A Frame of Reference for Health Knowledge

There is no necessary relationship between knowledge and health. Knowledge becomes purposeful in supporting health only by conscious intent. In order that knowledge may be acquired and utilized for the support of health, it is essential that a health problem be identified and the context of the application of the knowledge set forth as an hypothesis. From the discussion thus far, it is possible to identify the common loci for events that affect the state of health. Knowledge from each of these loci is necessary if the health problem is to be understood and resolved. The relative importance of improved knowledge from one or another of these loci will be dependent upon the nature of the health problem. At one extreme there is the complex, multi-factored issue of overpopulation and at the opposite extreme the presence of a disease such as infantile paralysis whose specific prevention by immunization epitomizes what applied knowledge of a unitary disease can accomplish.

A simplified frame of reference will place the common determinants of health and disease on one axis of a grid and the common points of application for effective change on an intersecting axis. The common determinants are:

1. Biologic events
2. Behavioral patterns
3. Economic conditions
4. Political organization
5. Institutional and organizational patterns for delivery
6. Cultural conditioning of the population
7. Ecologic system of which man is a part.

Knowledge and technology involving any or all of these common determinants may be applicable to any one or all of the following points of application for change:

1. Positive health maintenance
2. Specific disease prevention
3. Early specific diagnosis

4. Curative therapy
5. Supportive therapy
6. Rehabilitation training
7. Long-term supportive care.

To determine the adequacy of knowledge and the feasibility of applying it to any specific health problem it is necessary to identify the health problem within the frame of reference of the grid proposed above. One must then identify the critical path marked by the elements that place the effective limit on what can be accomplished by available efforts to remove the impediment to health.

In some conditions—for instance, specific metabolic diseases—the limiting factor may be predominately a deficit of biological knowledge and the technology potentially derived from it. In other problems, such as suicide or drug abuse, it is probable that limitations of knowledge in the behavioral sciences as well as a lack of feasible capacity to apply cultural and economic knowledge to a technology that would prevent suicide are more important. Knowledge for health is, therefore, not a single coherent field of study. It is, rather, the accumulation of information from a broad range of disciplines. The importance of biomedical research is beyond dispute but in recent decades there has been such an overweening awareness of it that the significance of other disciplines to health has been overshadowed.

Personal health services are based on knowledge that has feasible application. Of all available knowledge, both empirical and scientific, only a tiny fraction can now be applied to the technology of services. The whole realm of the humanities and arts falls almost completely outside this small fraction. At the opposite extreme the natural sciences have the highest probability of application to technology. It therefore occurs that even though a specific health problem might have its determinants in the economic and political realm—for instance, poverty-specific disease rates—the practical approach to these problems is probably not through increased knowledge of the economic and political factors. Rather, it requires a change in the actual economic and political conditions that created poverty in the first instance.

Because a disease state itself can usually be dealt with directly through applied biomedical information, one is likely to find that this feasibility is enough to establish a priority of effort to accumulate knowledge. In some instances this assumption of feasibility becomes generalized and dollars are invested in biological research on the faith that, through such basic research, knowledge will be obtained that will have sure feasibility of application to the technology necessary to resolve the problem. Under these circumstances, biomedical research has been heavily favored over research in the behavioral, cultural, institutional, and other determinants of health. This has been and will continue to be an essential strategy for the production of knowledge for health, but additional emphasis on research in the other determinants of health will be necessary in the future.

The Strategy of Biomedical Research

BASIC RESEARCH

Basic research, like beauty, is in the eye of the beholder. Characteristically, it is an investigation undertaken to satisfy the curiosity and interests of the investigator. In this context it can be understood as a branch of natural philosophy. The understanding of man's place in nature has been a human pursuit for as long as man has been conscious of his surroundings. This effort to improve understanding flows out of innate human curiosity and can be a highly lyrical form of creativity. It is no less an important expression of unpredictable creativity than literature, music, and the arts. It does not ask for justification beyond improved understanding, although it recognizes the frequent utility of such understanding. Although not confined to academic institutions, biological research as a branch of natural philosophy is more in the academic tradition than in the tradition of medicine itself. It is a form of human endeavor that requires continuing support if we are to continue our gradual improvement of understanding of man's nature.

Education at the professional level requires an environment that is zestful, questioning, and constantly seeking improvement. An essential element of this environment is a basic research program. Although applied research is also important, basic research is essential. An environment of basic research is best suited to display to the student the logic of scientific methodology. It is an antidote to the authoritarianism of a didactic and empirical approach to education. It continually stimulates in teacher and the student an attitude of rational skepticism about both fact and interpretation of fact. This not only substitutes enthusiasm for potential stagnation in the educational environment but it also prepares the student for the kind of continuing self-education that is the hallmark of the professional. It is hard to imagine but not inaccurate to assert that even though basic research efforts failed to improve understanding and had no application to practical affairs, they still would be justified as a central intellectual discipline for education in biology and medicine. Unfortunately, the support of basic research as an important component of the education of the Ph.D. and baccalaureate candidates as well as for the M.D. and other health professional candidates has been accidental rather than planned.

In practice, from 1945 to 1970 funds entering universities for support of biomedical research provided tremendous benefit to the quality of the educational environment as a side product. Unhappily, this has been accidental and to a degree illegal. With declining funds for the support of research, there is an adverse effect on educational programs. The opportunities for students to observe and participate in basic research are rapidly decreased as budgets are tightened, while the interest of students in entering a research career is aborted by the decreasing likelihood of support.

APPLIED RESEARCH

The term "applied research" is usually smeared with the implication of invidious comparison to basic research. Actually, research that has some purpose other than the purposes of natural philosophy and education falls under the heading of applied research. Closest to basic research is that applied research intended to provide feasible alternatives for choice. That is to say, there are many serious problems—for instance, cancer and arteriosclerosis—where we simply do not have fundamental information that allows us to make a choice about feasible approaches to effective control. The lack of such knowledge makes crash programs unavailable. Indeed, it is difficult to spend large sums of money wisely, with the exception of basic research funds, in these fields. A massive screening program of randomly derived chemical agents for possible therapeutic effect in cancer can waste almost unlimited amounts of money with no visible effect. Although one cannot predict what applied research aimed at producing effective chemotherapeutic agents may produce, at least it has a valid statistical likelihood of being productive. In fields such as mental health, culturally determined disorders, and disorders of destructive behavior, applied research is necessary in the loci of causation of these impediments to health. This kind of fundamental investigation is different from true basic research because it is the first step in programmed efforts to apply knowledge to technology designed to relieve a defined impediment to health.

Applied research that is more readily understood is either aimed at producing information specifically needed by desired technology or developing into technology basic information already produced. This is the research that is neatly programmed toward a specified intended change. It utilizes the same logic and technology as the most basic personal research that is contained in natural philosophy. In terms of rigor of intellectual discipline and sophistication of effort, it is in no sense less demanding than basic research. What is different is the purpose of the individual or group undertaking the effort. It was this kind of systematic research during the period of World War II that generated the general public awareness of the utility of knowledge in securing health. It is the kind of research most commonly found in private industry as well as being by far the greatest bulk of research supported by federal funds. It is important to understand, however, that this sort of research depends upon an underlying base of knowledge that is commonly produced either by the personal explorations of the natural philosopher or the fundamental investigator who is working in a field simply because it is likely to produce applicable knowledge even though the fruit of his efforts is unpredictable.

The Limitations of Biomedical Research

The importance of biomedical research to the health of mankind is so great that the uninformed now look upon it as a new magic capable of producing miracles at regular intervals. The promise of basic and applied biomedical research knowledge to further improvements of human health is so great that it titillates the imagination. As an antidote to unrealistic overenthusiasm, some comments are appropriate on the intrinsic limitations of this scientific discipline.

It has been possible through research to reduce complex living systems to smaller and smaller components that are manageable and can be examined in relatively simple cause-effect relationships. This reductionist approach has been the most productive research strategy in terms of understanding and effectiveness that has yet been devised. It gives us objective, quantitative, and reproducible descriptions instead of the intuitive and inexact observations inherent in empiricism. One of the most influential assumptions of modern biological science is that the very best and, indeed, the only truly scientific approach to the study of a natural phenomenon is to divide the living system into fragments and to investigate these elementary structures and their elementary properties. The danger in this assumption is that the reductionist approach may lead to a degree of emphasis on the elementary levels of organization of living systems that will divert concern for the actual phenomenon of human life which posed the question in the first instance.

At the present time it is not possible to provide a satisfying scientific description of so complex a phenomenon as a man. Our scientific descriptions are most convincing when they occur at an elemental level.

Even when we move to large, complex molecules, our degree of certainty is sharply decreased, and at the level of the cell and organ systems of life the certainty of scientific description is quite low. As complexity increases up to the final ecosystem we find that we are unable to predict events and, further, that the description of these phenomena in the physico-chemical terms which modern science uses is quite unsatisfying. The notion that physical concepts of causation which are valid at the molecular level will be applicable at the most complex level of organization of living systems remains to be convincingly demonstrated. This problem has been recognized in some areas and particularly in the field of genetics where the developing concern with population genetics now is offsetting the single-minded emphasis on molecular genetics that has captured the field for the last fifteen years.

Next to its limitations in dealing with high complexity, one of the most important limitations of biological research is the issue of uniqueness. At a very high statistical level of probability, each man is unique. Literature, art, and history are generally concerned with unique experiences. Science, on the other hand, deals with the unique only in terms of general principles. These general principles are derived from recurrent experiences which have a defined causal, logical explanation. Stated another way, as the indeterminacy of each cause-effect relationship is summated in the long chain of events that leads from molecule to man, the order of uncertainty becomes so high that the whole fabric of such a scientific explanation has very low validity, indeed. When one adds to this the observation that the interrelationships assumed causally in one man cannot be tested against an identical set in any other man, then the whole logic of exact scientific explanation of man is threatened.

We have already indicated that purposeful or applied research is sometimes fundamental but that much biomedical research falls in the realm of natural philosophy. Because basic research is without specific purpose other than the one that is self-justifying, it follows that such research cannot contribute to a value system derived from priorities of purpose. This is extremely important when we begin to make alternative choices based on scientific knowledge. That knowledge itself cannot actually provide the frame of reference in which the most valuable choice is made. There is broad, general awareness now that the human value of potential uses of scientific knowledge has to become an important part of the decision as to whether or not it should be produced in the first instance. This kind of value judgment falls outside of the realm of science.

Scientific knowledge is apolitical. Having access to the technology and substance of science does not provide the scientist with a preferred executive capacity in political decision making. The scientist has a special obligation to the political structure to inform, as best he can, of the likely outcome if one or another choice is made. On the other hand, it is not the natural prerogative of the scientist to be a central participant in that decision itself simply because he is a scientist. The disintegration of man as a social animal is threatened not only by the unplanned selective application of scientific research but in part by the very strategy of isolated scientific logic. The purposive intent for which that logic has no place is a necessary ingredient of political decisions if science itself is to serve humanistic health goals. Human values can become buried under an austere scientific discipline, and inappropriate technology forced on medicine in the name of society's need for scientific medicine. The primacy of the private, personal, subjective, individual experience that man has over any set of experiences of which science can now give a public and general account must be maintained as value-free and pure science continues to investigate the physicochemical explanations of living systems.

Opportunities for New Knowledge through Biomedical Research

In spite of its limitations and, indeed, of its dangers, biomedical research still remains the most promising single area for investment to produce new knowledge for health. From earlier portions of this discussion it is surely clear that other realms of research must be undertaken. On the other hand, it is also clear that fundamental and applied biological knowledge still remains the knowledge with the greatest feasible usefulness in improving man's health.

PROBLEMS OF INFECTION

Worldwide parasitic infections are the largest cause of death that is preventable. The basic principles of preventing, detecting, and treating infectious diseases are well understood. There remains, however, an urgent need for basic and developmental research to establish economically and politically feasible technologies for the control of parasitic diseases. The implications for such a concentrated effort are enormous. It has been estimated that the extension of schistosomiasis in the Egyptian population as the trematode extends into the impoundments of the Aswan Dam will create a new burden of disease that will come close to offsetting the total economic advantage of the dam. Twenty-five per cent of the population of Egypt suffers from bilharziasis, and the disease is widespread throughout the Orient. Malaria and sleeping sickness, amoebic dysentery and kala-azar are protozoan infections which, as a group, are still number one on the list of destroyers of human life. This single class of protozoan parasites does more than any other group of infectious organisms to reduce the significance of human life by making its survival unpredictable.

Viral diseases are not only annoying in the case of the common cold but deadly as well. Their relationship to cancer is evident but not well understood. Fundamental research into the nature of viral infection and disease is essential if we are to extend our technology of immunization and possibly chemotherapy against these deleterious agents.

NEOPLASTIC DISEASE

The variety of forms of neoplastic disease under the generic heading of cancer is beginning to be better understood. It appears now highly probable that the science of immunology is going to contain the essential ingredient which, added to our understanding of genetic predilection and environmental potentiation of the cancer-prone individual, will make feasible a technology not only of treatment but of prevention. Although some progress may be made in immuno-therapy and chemotherapy of neoplasms, it will not be until the feasibility of these strategies has been more firmly established through the development of fundamental knowledge that massive efforts will be justified. There is probably no field of medicine in which knowledge moves more rapidly from the laboratory to the patient than in the field of cancer. There is also probably no other field in which the variety and depth of fundamental research required are as great in order to produce effective knowledge.

ATHEROSCLEROSIS

The origins of arterial occlusion associated with accumulation of fatty deposits under the lining of the blood vessels are not well understood. It is probable that the causation is multiple and that no single factor is controlling. On the other hand, it appears likely that a consistent part of the disorder is the accumulation of cholesterol and lipids. Where the blood level of cholesterol is high, this accumulation is enhanced, although it may occur in the absence of significantly elevated blood cholesterol levels. It is also clear that hypertension is an important participating element in the rate of focal development of these fatty deposits.

Both cholesterol metabolism and hypertension have now been defined well enough so that a major investment in developmental research has a high probability of producing therapeutic agents that will significantly control the occurrence of heart disease and stroke caused by occlusive atherosclerosis. There is no doubt that eating and living habits contribute to the problems. But it is not clear what information can be added to effect a change in these habits that would be as effective as the potential change created by the development of therapeutic agents that are now theoretically feasible.

CONTRACEPTION AND ABORTION

If the so-called population explosion is to be contained, there must be a decrease in the desirability of having children in excessive numbers, by changes in economic, cultural, and religious values. The knowledge for producing this value change is uncertain in origin and unpredictable in application. Meantime it seems plausible at least to provide readily available means for preventing the conception or birth of unwanted children. The physiology of the onset of menstruation and of the onset of labor is not now well enough understood so that highly specific contraceptive and abortifacient agents are available. Although oral contraceptives have been extraordinarily effective in interrupting the normal menstrual cycle and placing it under extraneous hormonal control, the need for daily ingestion of medication and the multiplicity of side effects make it something less than an ideal approach. In the same manner, there is now no well established physiologic abortifacient. In the early weeks of pregnancy the only available and reliable technique is a mechanical or chemical evacuation of the uterine contents. There is no theoretical reason why an improved knowledge of the mechanism of the onset of labor and the induction of menstruation could not lead to the development of a physiologic abortifacient which would greatly simplify and expedite the early termination of an unwanted pregnancy.

The development of an oral contraceptive agent for men has had only very limited study, but the complex set of stages in spermatogenesis is as readily available for interruption as the series of physiologic events in the female menstrual cycle.

The point of this discussion of abortion is that we are at a stage where fundamental knowledge gives high promise of success in research productivity for the development of more convenient and physiologic contraceptive and abortifacient agents. For the immediate future this would appear to be the only assured means of controlling somewhat the excessive growth of population throughout the world.

PROBLEMS OF PRIORITY

In considering these opportunities for biomedical research no attempt has been made to be exhaustive or to discuss in significant detail the specific diseases or health problems. Rather, it is intended to emphasize that the present national priorities for limitation of research are terribly misguided. This is so because there is close to hand available knowledge through research that will make tremendous contributions to human health. There can surely be debate about whether we should invest large amounts of money in developing knowledge aimed at genetic engineering or test tube babies, because the social utility of these is obscure. It would, however, be tragic to fail to take advantage of the availability of knowledge clearly essential for health that biomedical research can provide.

Conclusion as to Biomedical Research

Health is a state free of impediment to the fulfillment of human potential. Any condition that limits human purpose limits health. Any knowledge that contributes to our capacity for self-fulfillment contributes to health.

Knowledge for health is a part of natural philosophy, is essential to the educational process, and is the foundation of changed practices that will improve personal health service.

Of the many realms of knowledge which are significant to health, the most promising for our generation is the utility of knowledge produced by biomedical research. Biomedical research is in itself insufficient as an approach to health knowledge and has many intrinsic limitations. Support of biomedical research alone will not produce the variety of knowledge necessary to solve man's problems of health. On the other hand, it is probable that the highest public benefit from resources invested with the purpose of improving health will be, for some years to come, the multiple payoffs of knowledge derived from biomedical research.

Education for Health Knowledge in Action

It has been estimated (1968 Health Resources Statistics publication, *Public Health Service*) that 3.4 million persons were employed in 1967 in the health professions and occupations, divided into 21 categories of full-time workers. This represented four per cent of the total civilian labor force and sixteen per cent of all professional and technical workers in the United States. Of this number, there were 294,000 M.D. physicians (Doctor of Medicine) and another 11,400 D.O. physicians (Doctor of Osteopathy). In addition to 660,000 registered nurses, there were an additional 1,130,000 practical nurses, nurse aides, and home health aides. A survey at The University of Michigan in 1968 showed that there were 88 formal educational programs leading to specific health related occupations. The logistics for the education of this remarkable variety and number of full-time health workers is such a formidable problem that without an increased efficiency in the utilization of the existing work force, it is highly improbable that the expectations of the nation for delivery of health services can be met.

The National Advisory Commission on Health Manpower in 1967 suggested that the health industry would become the nation's largest employer by 1975. They came face to face with the paradox that while the number of physicians, hospital beds, and health services per person were generally equal to or greater than 30 years ago, the social utility of new medical knowledge and the growth of purchasing power from private and public insurance programs have increased demand for services until there is truly a health care crisis. This, however, is not simply a crisis of numbers. Although substantially increased numbers will be needed over time, unless we improve the system itself there will continue to be a discrepancy between productive capacity and demands, even though there are massive increases in costs of units of services and in numbers of health care personnel.

BACKGROUND OF MEDICAL EDUCATION

The present status of medical education in the United States and the changes it is undergoing require some historical perspective if they are to be understood. During its colonial period, America did not have formally organized medical schools, and clergymen with some medical knowledge were the chief medical practitioners along with a few apprentices of physicians trained in Europe and in England.

It was John Morgan in 1765 at the University of Pennsylvania who was responsible for the first medical school north of Mexico, and it was he who, in his "Discourse upon the Institution of Medical Schools in America," set forth the principles which are still valid today. These principles have their derivation from the classical period of Hippocratic medicine, through its renaissance at Padua and its statement around the turn of the eighteenth century at the University of Leiden in Holland by Boerhaave. His concern that the patient should be the object of instruction, but that bedside impressions should be examined by pathological studies so that the science and the art of medicine could reinforce each other, still stands today.

Medicine is still engaged in the application of scientific knowledge to human purposes. It is the physician who stands as the personification of this effort. If the purpose of medical education is to be fulfilled, the physician must fulfill himself through dedicated service to the art and the science of medicine for the good of his patient. John Monroe, who was a student of Boerhaave, carried these traditions to establish the great medical school at Edinburgh. From Edinburgh and from the hospital schools of London there flowed to North America the traditions established by Boerhaave in Leiden. Toward the end of the nineteenth century, William Osler studied medicine at McGill University in Canada and then moved to the University of Pennsylvania before becoming the first professor of medicine at Johns Hopkins University. It was the Johns Hopkins medical school which served as the prototype model by which all medical schools in the United States were judged in the Flexner study, 1908–1910.

Medical education had got off to a good start in the United States, so that the five medical schools existing in 1790 all had university sponsorship. Between 1800 and 1860 a new medical school was started about every year, most of them unrelated to a university. It was only in 1851 that salaried professorships for medical faculty were first established by a state university—The University of Michigan. By the end of the Civil War only 46 medical schools remained in the United States, but in the succeeding 30 years the total rose to 160, most of which were run as private enterprises by medical practitioners and had no standard curriculum or academic discipline. In 1900 less than ten per cent of those practicing medicine in the United States were graduates of any regular medical school.

The relative handful of university associated medical schools, along with the more responsible practitioners in the United States, began to work toward establishing national standards for medical education. Between 1875 and 1908, the American Medical Association and the Association of American Medical Colleges led this battle, which culminated in 1908 when the Carnegie Foundation for the Advancement of Teaching supported the famous study by Abraham Flexner, who was himself a teacher of classics. This revolution of the early century represents the new rigidity; and medical education in the United States is in the process of breaking away from the patterns epitomized by the Flexner Report.

PRESENT STATE OF MEDICAL EDUCATION

Medical education in the United States is characterized by four separate but interrelated phases:

Preprofessional education of the future physician is the responsibility of the college faculty of liberal arts and sciences and extends over a period of four years, which represents the thirteenth through sixteenth years of formal schooling. The student completing his four years of liberal arts college is about 21 years old when he enters the medical school.

Professional education at the level of M.D. candidacy is the unique responsibility of the faculty of medicine. For over 50 years the curriculum in the United States has been a 4-year sequence. So-called basic medical sciences are emphasized in the first 2 years; the clinical sciences with their patient-centered learning dominate the last 2.

Postdoctoral education is based in the hospital and is the responsibility of the medical staff. The first year after the M.D. degree has historically been called an *internship;* subsequent years are called *residency.* The average formal hospital training after graduation lasts from four to five years.

Postgraduate education continues throughout the physician's practice and is largely an individual obligation. Increasingly, professional societies and medical schools are providing organized instruction for practitioners as an integral part of their educational programs.

For many years these four phases have been separate from each other. Recently emphasis has been placed on the advantage of integrating them. Within the curriculum of the medical school there has been, for over 30 years, a continuing effort to erase the unnatural segregation of medical education into basic and clinical phases. The unity of the full program of professional education of the physician is now axiomatic and is a reference standard for evolving curriculum and administration.

Since community hospitals attract the majority of medical graduates for intern and residency training, the postdoctoral period of medical education usually is apart from the faculties of medical schools. Even within those hospitals that are integrated or fully affiliated with medical schools, only a tentative beginning has been made to associate intern and residency training with the academic responsibility of the medical school. Within all hospitals, the rotating internship that was designed for all new graduates is slowly giving way to a blending of the internship and residency into a continuum appropriate for the final form of practice.

The Medical Center

The intrinsic unity of the education of a physician creates powerful forces directed toward a coordinated educational program extending from the high school through the continuing practice. Such a program requires in its professional phase the environment of a medical center. The center must embody the university ideal of academic freedom in a scholarly community that is responsible for medical research, medical teaching, and the care of patients. The medical center itself is a complex providing resources as nearly comprehensive as can be achieved. Its core units are a medical school, associated research laboratories and a hospital integrated with the medical school along with its outpatient facilities.

Education in nursing and dentistry commonly utilizes the medical center resources as do many of the programs for related health workers in fields such as physical therapy, clinical psychology, medical social work, medical technology, and many others. Schools of public health have typically been established in a university medical center setting; in their absence, the medical school and hospital must assume a direct concern with the problems of public health practice, teaching, and research. Most university medical centers today have, in addition, specialized units for research and clinical care. These may be separate institutes or, more commonly, they are incorporated within the departments of the school and hospital. They reflect educational interests at the postdoctoral level as well as special institutional capabilities in research. The size and content of the university medical center is controlled by available resources—in operating funds, buildings, supply of patients and, most importantly, its ability to attract faculty and students of excellence. The presence of vigorous and imaginative leadership is essential to such a university medical center.

The System of Medical Education

The changes in medical education in the United States have many things in common with those of other countries of the world, but their particular form is shaped by the society of which they are a part and which they must serve. American medicine and medical education are evolving under the influence of unprecedented demands for service and the force of expanding scientific knowledge. The stresses of accelerating rates of change have created a seeming paradox: a widespread discontent with the entire system of medical research, teaching, and clinical service at a time when the quality and magnitude of each of these components are at the highest level ever achieved. Rising costs and shortages of physicians, dentists, nurses, and other health professionals have rasied serious doubts as to whether the "system" as it is now constituted can meet the quantitative demand and at the same time rapidly deliver to the public the advantages of increasing scientific knowledge. The re-emergence of proprietary schools outside the jurisdiction of the university is a likelihood if those now responsible for medical education fail to meet these quantitative needs.

When only doctors were responsible for patient care, concern with delivery of health service could be contained and defined. The idea of the physician as a private entrepreneur has heavily influenced the growth of a segregated curriculum. Medical education has been a leader in establishing standards that justify this professional status. These same educational standards are now being widely copied in each of the related health professions, and each seeks a degree of professional identity and independence analogous to that of the physician. When the education of nurses and dentists was added about 100 years ago to the American universities, the advantages of a separate identity for their curricula were compelling. At the present time in our history, however, the increase in the number of medically related specialists trained at all academic levels recreates the ancient problems of the Tower of Babel.

There is no mechanism that attempts to relate precisely the variety of educational programs to the actual needs of the community. Since only the university can contain the broad range of research and education necessary to the total "system" of health services, there is a need for the university to address itself to this same "system" of health-related education, research, and organization. Still if self-determination is to remain a hallmark of the medical profession, then that profession must assume more effective leadership in these changing times. The faculties of medicine have a particular responsibility of achieving the highest level possible within the present system while preparing themselves and their students for an uncertain but surely changed future.

The principles guiding the evolution of the medical school curriculum in the United States are: (1) to provide for a greater flexibility of the medical school curriculum; (2) to give increased emphasis to the relevance of theoretical material to the problems of human health and disease from the beginning; and (3) to try to shorten the time utilized in the formal education of the physician.

The Health Manpower Shortage

The simple question of whether there is a physician shortage could be answered by an equally simple *yes*. If the question is changed, however, to ask what *degree* of physician shortage we have in the United States, then it is not possible to give an exact answer.

The fact of a shortage is not beyond dispute. The ratio of physicians to population in the United States has been approximately constant for well over 30 years. In this time the general burden of illness has decreased and longevity has increased. The United States has a comparatively higher physician population ratio than England or the European and Scandinavian countries. There are over twice as many surgeons in ratio to population in the United States as there are in England, while only half as many operations are performed in England. The morbidity and mortality data of the United States and England insofar as surgical disorders are concerned are not different. The citizens of the United States make more frequent use of physicians than in most western countries—approximately 50 per cent greater utilization than in Great Britain.

Every medical school in the United States admits its full quota of students. The academic qualifications of entering students are at the highest level of history, while the ratio of applicants to places available has not changed substantially in fifteen years. In spite of all this, it is probably true that we do have a serious shortage of physicians and that the shortage will grow more pressing in the future.

The output of new graduates from American medical schools is nearly 2,000 a year short of keeping pace with the rate of growth of the population. This difference has been made up since the early forties by the immigration of an equivalent number of graduates of foreign medical schools. It is probable that the United States should, instead, be exporting physicians to countries seriously under-supplied, and it is certainly not in the national interest to have a physician production system that requires a large number of foreign graduates each year in order to maintain a traditional physician-population ratio.

Less than half of the approved residency positions in American hospitals are filled by American graduates. There are twice as many internship positions offered each year in the hospitals of the United States as can be filled by graduates from American medical schools. From the point of view of our hospitals, therefore, there is no doubt that a very real shortage exists in physician supply.

Medical education in the United States has not responded adequately to the desire of qualified students to enter the study of medicine. Historically, about two students apply for each place in the entering class of the nation's medical schools. In recent years this number has increased slightly, but more important, the qualifications of the applicants have strikingly improved. The result is that because of a limited number of places, *qualified* students are more and more frequently excluded. This opportunity problem is heightened when one observes the very small number of medical students whose social and economic advantages are at or below the national averages. It is, of course, true that this failure of opportunity to study medicine occurs initially at the point of entrance into college, but it is further expressed in an effective lack of opportunity to go to medical school. This lack of equal access for all qualified students is at the root of an inadequate system of producing physicians.

Since 1965, the number of students entering medical schools has increased by approximately 500 to a level of 9,700 in 1969. By 1972 it is anticipated that approximately 11,000 students will be entering if the present plans for all the new and existing medical schools are funded. This latter condition will not be met at the present rate of new funding. It is therefore certain that the shortage of physicians will continue in the United States for at least the next ten years. Medical students entering in the fall of 1970 will graduate in 1974 and will spend an average of four years in hospital-based training after which the vast majority can look forward to two years of military duty, thus entering community practice in 1980.

If the discrepancy between demand and supply is to be reduced within the next ten to fifteen years, then it must be through an improved organization in delivery of health services while every effort is made to increase the total number of entering medical students and to shorten the duration of their total training period. The hospital is the inevitable focus of efforts to improve the efficiency of physician utilization and the education of the physician. Historically, medical school curricula were developed with the notion that graduates were prepared to enter general practice, sometimes after a year of internship but many times in the past without such a hospital experience. Now, it would be more accurate to say that the function of a medical school curriculum is to prepare the new graduate for an equal number of years of hospital-based education.

Community hospitals are now the focal point of health services and are the place where physicians and other health related clinical practitioners concentrate. The hospital, therefore, has evolved from being simply a place where physicians worked to an institution that is an integral part of the production of physicians. It is the principal social institution for the coordination and distribution of health services. University hospitals stand now on the threshold of a new era of responsibility. This responsibility is to demonstrate that the quality, effectiveness, cost, and availability of health services can be improved to the point where the expectations of the people are met. Just as the university hospitals made themselves models for the demonstration of how scientific knowledge can be introduced into and modify the practice of medicine, so now they must look forward to efforts in research and education that will optimize the utilization of physicians and health related professionals.

The shortage of physicians is expressed as a discrepancy between demand and supply of physician services. The capacity to supply services will be met only in part by an increase in the number of physicians. Of equal importance, and hopefully more immediately available, are organizational solutions to the problems of economy and effectiveness made possible by a reorganization of the delivery of health services. The final test of our educational programs, for all health professions and allied health occupations, is whether through them the health of the people is served to the fullest capacity of scientific knowledge and human dedication.

James L. Goddard

5

Health Protection

On August 6, 1945, an American B-29 dropped an atomic bomb on Hiroshima, Japan, a city of 245,000. The burst sucked up most of the city in a column of smoke and debris 50,000 feet high. The fireball was a half-mile wide. Eighty thousand lives went into that mushroom cloud. Another 100,000 persons suffered injuries. Nearly all of the city's 200 doctors and 1,800 nurses were killed or injured during the blast and the ensuing firestorm. The Japanese, first victims of the atomic age, next lost the city of Nagasaki before suing for peace and the end of World War II.

On March 1, 1954, the United States inaugurated the age of fission-fusion-fission by setting off the first hydrogen bomb from the test platform on the Bikini Atoll. A 23-man Japanese fishing vessel, the *Lucky Dragon*, accidentally wandered into the fallout zone. It was covered with the light gray radioactive ash. Radioman Aikichi Kuboyama died on September 23 and his own ashes were placed in a vault on the hillside overlooking the port city of Yaizu. The Japanese, first victims of the hydrogen age, were paid $2 million by the American government for this tragedy.

It is probably better to leave history alone, to shunt these events

JAMES L. GODDARD, M.D., *former commissioner of the Food and Drug Administration, has been assistant surgeon general of the U.S. Public Health Service, civil air surgeon of the Federal Aviation Agency, and chief of the Communicable Disease Center in Atlanta. Contributor of many articles to professional journals, Dr. Goddard is now vice president of EDP Technology, Inc., of Atlanta, and is under temporary contract to the Ford Foundation program of assistance to the Government of India in population control.*

deeper into footnotes, and search out new things, the discoveries of today and the portents for tomorrow. Yet history repeats itself—how well man has learned that lesson—and, as Santayana observed, those who ignore history are doomed to relive it.

For Americans concerned about the development of health protection, a number of questions arise, questions posed—and, since then, partially explained and answered—by the atomic and hydrogen bomb explosions:

1. How broad an assignment of responsibility should scientists and technologists assume and how should they be educated and trained for it?
2. If priorities in research are to be set, what criteria should be used to discover them?
3. What are the end-points in planning; how precise and how close-in should the objectives of planning be?
4. If man is to be the beneficiary of developments in health protection, how do we prevent his becoming the first innocent, violated object of those very developments?

The Fermis, Einsteins, Tellers, and Oppenheimers had "nothing to do with" the doctors of Hiroshima or the fisherman of Yaizu. Or did they? Their tasks were circumscribed, in that the development of the bomb was the first order of business—and the last as well. The possible range of "fallout" from their bombs—biological, ecological—was confined within a parochial plan (parochial in hindsight, we must admit). And the arguments of risk-to-benefit have all been post facto, giving us very little understanding of the true nature of these physical science discoveries and how to use them wisely.

During the last third of the twentieth century, Americans are beginning to grapple with some of the basic questions of human survival, even as they hold the power to destroy humanity itself. To ignore all this as the context for a discussion of health and mechanisms of health protection would deprive that very discussion of its motive power. While some elements may be a good deal less awesome than the fireball raised above the Bikini Atoll, the issues and the questions do join; the world must be seen whole, as the sum of interlocking parts.

The Resources for Protection

PROFESSIONAL, TECHNICAL, AND LAY MANPOWER

Overall, the appearance of research and development manpower —scientists and engineers primarily—is accelerating: the growth rate for this group has been better than seven per cent annually, compared to less than two per cent annual growth rate for the labor force as a whole. These rates represent the early and middle years of the decade of the sixties, years during which research and development were given very substantial financial support in both the public and private sectors, making this an attractive career choice. Regardless of the fluctuation in such support for the years that follow on, the R&D manpower produced during the early and middle sixties represents a substantial component from which the field of health may draw.

This is particularly appropriate when discussing health protection, since protective—or preventive—health activity is multidisciplinary, requiring the contributions of physicians, medical researchers, and engineers and physical scientists as well. If we take this broad view of manpower with *potential* contributions to health, we can speak of a pool of a half-million scientists and engineers, among whom are many with direct or indirect ties to human health. These half-million R&D personnel link up with about 300,000 physicians, 900,000 nurses (registered and licensed practical nurses), and nearly 100,000 dentists. To these we might add about 125,000 pharmacists and another 150,000 or so "allied health" personnel, non-professional but increasingly effective.

If we pool all these manpower categories and consider them all as appropriate for a role in health protection, we come up with about one per cent of the nation's population. When we consider that dentists fix engineers' teeth and nurses take care of sick engineers, the availability of health personnel to the general public is further limited.

Health Protection as Professional Career Choice—But putting aside statistics for a moment, there is yet another and far more significant problem to consider regarding manpower for health protection: how are these scientific, engineering, medical, and health personnel trained to see the world of health care? The general answer would be this: as reparative or curative personnel. For the most part, the engineers in the health field are occupied with the development of artificial hearts, lungs, kidneys, and so on. The medical instrumentation coming upon the scene is reflective of the preoccupation most health professionals exhibit with repairing damages, curing diseases, and replacing parts.

Why does a heart suddenly stop? Why does a kidney fail? These are extremely difficult questions. Researchers have devoted professional lifetimes to seeking answers and have experienced the giving out of their own hearts before making *the* definitive contribution to an answer. Such self-effacement is simply not attractive to many young professionals, who would rather aim their careers toward some tangible achievements. This is understandable. And it is possible to design and construct an artificial kidney or a heart pacemaker or a synthetic artery within one's lifetime.

The motivation for most of the manpower in the health field does not coincide with the needs of the field of health protection and disease prevention. Fulfillment, in terms of monetary or psychic income, is heavily weighted on the side of reparative and curative medicine. Schools of medicine, nursing, engineering, and dentistry reveal this all too clearly in their course catalogs, not to mention in the careers of their graduates.

Nonprofessional Lay Health Worker—The demand, however, is quite clearly growing for better mechanisms to provide protection for the human, to prevent the occurrence of illness, disease, and stress. If the professional and technical community has not reordered its own priorities to meet this demand, who then steps forth? The nonprofessional. Surely one of the most important phenomena of current events in the health field is the appearance and rapid development of the lay health worker. The titles or job descriptions are indicative of the range of activity and the kind of demand being met: physicians' aides, home health care workers, family counselors, health educators, nursing aides, health administrators, associate therapists, dental assistants and dental aides, dispensary technicians, etc. The health career field has been greatly enlarged, reaching into education, law, and the behaviorial sciences, with the accent being heavily on the kinds of training, experience, and inclination that lead to protecting the health of the individual, rather than solely on restoring it after it has been impaired or lost.

Informed Consumer as Health Protector—The last category of "health manpower" which is becoming increasingly important is the informed consumer. The more the individual understands the requirements of his physical and mental well-being, the more effectively does he participate in the health system. The popular press—all the mass media—provide the lay public with the interest to learn more about both the nature of the health care problem and the ways it can be relieved. Through such popularizations (acknowledging all their shortcomings, oversimplifications, false promises, and so on), the consumer does gain a higher level of understanding and a certain facility for identifying danger, stress, or other kinds of insults, and for heading the other way.

We might fret about the lack of enthusiasm with which the smoking public is giving up cigarettes; but those who guide the tobacco industry have not been fooled: they have been extremely busy diversifying into other industries (principally food processing). Similarly, after a period of time, the public has begun to look for safety features in automobiles; they are convinced that seat belts work, that it is preferable to have a seat belt lying on your abdomen than a piece of steering wheel lodged in your lung.

The growth rate of health manpower on an annual basis is slightly above that of the population in general. But the demand for more services from the general population far exceeds the response possible even by a larger pool of health professionals. Hence, the perimeters of the field have been generously thrown open, even to including the informed consumer as a member of the health team active in protection and preventive medicine.

RESEARCH AND NEW KNOWLEDGE

The best that can be said about the development of new information in the health field is that it has been modest. Approximately 4 per cent of the total health bill for 1968—about $54 billion—was devoted to research. Much of that research, however, represents a refinement of data and techniques that already exist. For example, in the field of dentistry, there are various predictions for the expansion of dental care in the future. By 1980 as many as 20 million children whose families would not have been able to afford the dental care of the 1960s will be receiving such care, according to some health economists. By that year the revolution in high-speed painless drilling (or sonic drilling or whatever) will have been completed. Power-operated floor equipment—stools, chairs, cabinets, etc.—will be at hand as well. The United States Department of Commerce is already keeping its eye on such things as "ultrasonic cleaners, autoclaves, and sterilizers, as well as on better illumination such as the use of concentrated beam for lighting oral cavities." The department continues, "Intensive research is being carried on for a material which will withstand rejection when dentures are implanted. At present," the department wrote in 1968, "cobalt crystal appears to be promising. Another technological advance which will spur the growth of the industry appears to be the bonding of porcelain to acrylic. Porcelain bonding to gold for crowns and cap will also increase because of its cosmetic value as well as durability."

In other words, for much of the research—in both the public and private sectors—in the field of dentistry it is pretty much business as usual, but possibly more so. Dentistry is probably the most obvious specialty within the health field in which reparative work, reparative philosophies, training, research, and industrial support are so evident.

Yet, dentistry, while prominent on this score, is assuredly not alone. Therefore, when we speak of the development of new knowledge through research for improving the course of health protection, we may tend to speak wistfully.

New Body of Knowledge Needed—Unfortunately, the decade of the sixties has alerted us only to certain hard-core areas of research that have to be penetrated. It has not proved to be the decade of the great breakthroughs. This may be argued in just one special area: molecular biology and the synthesis of deoxyribonucleic acid (DNA). Considering the significance of unlocking, as it were, the genetic code embedded within DNA and RNA (ribonucleic acid) in the very heart of the nucleus of the human cell, the estimated several millions spent on this single area of research in 1968 is embarrassingly small.

It is, of course, unfair to dismiss the efforts of our research community as being of small value. That is not true. Thousands of man-years are consumed within our great medical research centers by projects that do contribute in large measure to the physical and mental well-being of the population. However, the research designs are still drawn with known data as reference points. Essentially, our medical and health research is improving upon the corpus of knowledge we already have. That is fine. But we also need—and need desperately—a corpus of new information with few known reference points.

Seven Anchor Points for New Health Planning—In 1965, E. R. Weinerman described what he called the new "Anchor Points Underlying the Planning for Tomorrow's Health Care." These anchor points actually approach man and his disease conditions from a different, unconventional point of view. Weinerman lists these as his points of departure tomorrow:

1. Known elements of risks, including environmental conditions.
2. Complex etiology; in fact, multiple causes are the rule rather than the exception in diagnostics today.
3. Non-preventability, which accepts the human, contemporary condition and many of its distinct and oppressive—and permanent—aspects.
4. Non-specificity, an anchor point related to the etiological problem.
5. Multiple manifestations, a phenomenon that has already jarred the art of diagnostics and continues to confuse the drug therapist.
6. Impaired social function, a condition that draws the physician or the treatment team into a wide arena of exploration.
7. Chronicity—the phenomenon of illness just not going away.

These seven points are quite general, somewhat vague, definitely unsettling. They do not conform to the accepted outline of "what's wrong with people today." Which is precisely Weinerman's point.

Whether or not he has chosen the most relevant anchor points for tomorrow's health planner is meat for discussion. Nevertheless, as we continue to invest in research and the development of new knowledge, these seven points take on increased meaning.

Illustrating Application of Anchor Points—Once again, these anchor points bring to mind the ordeal of Aikichi Kuboyama. The American team that detonated the Bikini H-bomb was aware of most of the elements of risk—but not all of them, to be sure. Even the wind direction on that March day in the Pacific was misjudged. Kuboyama might still be alive and fishing had all or even most of the elements of risk been calculated prior to detonation.

Kuboyama was given massive transfusions of blood so that the ultimate cause of his death was never really determined. An acute liver disorder, probably brought on by serum hepatitis carried in the plasma, has been given as the primary cause of his death. On the other hand, the degeneration of his liver has been attributed to the "debris" of cells injured or destroyed by radiation. Finally, he was judged by many to have died as a result of simple radiation injury.

The nuclear physicist Ralph Lapp, who became personally involved in the case of the *Lucky Dragon* and its doomed radioman, said later, "The fact remains that the cause of Kuboyama's death will probably never be known with certainty, but if he had not been dusted with the radioactive ash he would never have needed a blood transfusion. Thus the argument about the cause of his death was rather pointless." This is, one might say, a conclusion more political than medical. Today, medicine is challenged by such "pointless" arguments concerning the etiology of illness and disease.

The course of history tends to be all-engulfing, overwhelming. Despite the comments a few paragraphs above that the detonation team ought to have known more of the elements of risk than they did know, it is clear that the bomb was to have been detonated on March 1 willy-nilly and it is also clear that the *Lucky Dragon* would not go to the Solomon Islands to fish but would head toward Midway—since the fishing conditions dictated that change of direction.

For several days the sickness that came over the crew was not exactly identified. But these were the symptoms: nausea, itching skin, irritated eyes, some fever, diarrhea, listlessness, darkening of the skin, and falling hair. By the time they reached Yaizu, the suspicions were quite strong: they had the "atomic sickness." Finally, Geiger counters made specific what had been an uneasy, non-specific suspicion for several days.

Weinerman's fifth, sixth, and seventh "anchor points" have antecedents in the experience of the *Lucky Dragon*'s crew; there is no need to belabor the idea. What needs to be emphasized, however, is that health protection—protecting the health of the human through better delivery of care by professionals who have better training and are supplied with better information—is still a hope. We have a limited supply of irrelevantly trained people who operate in an obsolete treatment environment supported by research on the old questions. That is a harsh but very possibly the most honest statement we can make as we enter the final third of the most exciting and still the most perplexing century in the history of man.

The Nature of Protection

The concept of protection has implicit within it the elements of attack upon something—in the case of this discussion, the human organism. The human is under intensive attack; to describe these attacks and the ways to protect against them requires some framework, no matter how arbitrary, or else the whole discussion collapses into scattershot. We can look at health protection, therefore, as it affects the human in three environments: *personal, immediate,* and *general.* This is a reasonable—albeit arbitrary—arrangement and gives us an opportunity to segregate our data and our logic for greater comprehension.

THE PERSONAL ENVIRONMENT

The personal environment is, literally, an internal matter. The contemporary human is surrounded by an estimated 250,000 different chemical substances, many of which he eats, drinks, or inhales, with or without his full knowledge. These so-called "insults" to the human organism are not completely understood, since many of the substances have been introduced since the 1940s; a full generation of men and women has not yet experienced the total effect of these substances.

Even as this ignorance is acknowledged, the continued and expanded use of all types of drugs goes on. The "drug explosion" of the 1950s, coming hard on the heels of the antibiotics revolution of World War II, is still reverberating. There are approximately 21,000 different drug products in the American marketplace. These products are based on about 7,000 different chemicals (single entities or combinations of chemical entities). We may consider ourselves fortunate; one country of Western Europe is reported to have 55,000 drug products available to consumers, doubling the order of magnitude of our problem in America.

Extent of Drug Use—When the subject of drugs is raised, most individuals respond with such terms as *LSD, pot, bennies,* and *goofballs*. These are drugs, or the street name for drugs (lysergic acid diethylamide, marijuana, stimulants, depressants, respectively), that have a potential for abuse and are clearly a danger to the consumer. This is an opportunity to launch into a lengthy essay on drug abuse, but such an essay would concern itself with a minority of the population. We should be more concerned with the majority of the population who ingest drugs of all kinds—prescription and nonprescription— at an incredible rate.

In 1968, an international symposium on the physiology and pathology of sleep was informed that one out of four persons in America uses a sedative of some kind to induce sleep. And the figure is rising as surveys and sampling techniques reach deeper into the population. One member of the conference said that about 14 per cent of the population suffered from insomnia; yet, 25 per cent were trying to go to sleep with the aid of drugs. Doctors prescribe barbiturates— sodium pentobarbital was the most popular in a Los Angeles survey of 102 physicians—although few are aware of the effects of barbiturates upon the human. The drugs will put a person to sleep; that is true enough. But they also produce undesirable symptoms, such as psychic and physical dependence, impaired motor coordination, and even psychotic responses (suicide attempts, etc.).

"Better living through chemistry," the slogan of one of the country's major chemical corporations, was taken up by the "hippie" colony in San Francisco's Haight-Asbury section. But in the suburbs of Marin County, down in Redwood City, in Palo Alto, Salinas, and Monterey, across to Phoenix, Salt Lake City, and straight east to Kennebunkport, the reach for chemistry by the average American has been prodigious. In 1968, the one-billion-prescription mark was topped as an annual figure: a billion prescriptions for 200 million people.

The largest single drug group is the antibiotic, used for colds, fevers, chronic illnesses, infections, and other diseases. The next cluster of heavily prescribed drugs includes tranquilizers, oral contraceptives, and heart drugs. The first is taken to help the modern man or woman cope with contemporary life; the second is the answer to two problems: mechanical inhibitions on the sex act and the production of unwanted children; the third reflects, essentially, the increased longevity we seem to have attained (we picked up about two years between 1950 and 1970; current life expectancy for today's infants is age 70 or slightly better) and the development, since 1966, of broadscale programs to aid the aging, such as Medicare and Medicaid. The elderly (over-65) Americans account for about 200 million prescriptions a year —well over $800 million worth of drugs—which is a good indication of where the succeeding generations are heading: more of the same. In the mid-1960s, a survey team from the Stanford Research Institute found that 86 "typically American" households had 2,539 medications on hand, or a mean of 29.5 per household. A sixth were prescription; the rest were nonprescription drugs. They were in medicine cabinets, bureau drawers, and kitchen trays, ready to treat everything from poison ivy to stomach "gas" to diabetes. The prevalence of drugs in the home—right at hand for young and old—is a significant indicator of the kind of chemical assault taking place within the human, in his own personal environment.

Increasing Use of Food Additives—Add to the drug intake the ingestion of food additives—about 3.5 pounds of such chemistry a year, out of a total per capita food intake of 1,000 pounds. Is this a little or a lot? No one is sure. Some of the additives, such as salt, pepper, and talc, have been with us for a long time, but not studied. Others, such as the flavoring agent 2-hexyl-4-acetoxytetrahydrofuran, are fairly new and not studied with any real depth before being placed in general use, nor studied at all after general usage is approved (food additives, like drugs, enter the marketplace only after receiving the approval of the federal government). In 1955 the U.S. population consumed about 419 million pounds of additives; by 1966, the figure jumped nearly 60 per cent to 661 million pounds; for 1975, the estimate (by Arthur D. Little, Inc.) is 1.03 billion pounds of food additives. These rises in food additive usage are completely inconsistent with population increases or other conventional indicators: there are always more people eating more food. But the evidence seems to show that more people will eat more food containing much more chemical manipulation that ever before.

Interaction of Drugs and Food Additives—Ordinarily there should be no cause for concern. Except that we are arriving at one of those "anchor points" described by Weinerman. We are already witnessing drug-and-drug and drug-and-food interactions that are harmful and, thus far, not always predictable. Here are some examples:

1. Antibacterial or antifungal agents, such as Furazolidone, Griseofulvin, the Sulfanamides, and the Tetracyclines, interact with alcohol, phenobarbital, aspirin, methanamine, collodial antacids, milk, and other dairy products.
2. Antidiabetic agents interact with alcohol, aspirin, and other salicyclates.
3. Antihypertensive agents react with alcohol, antihistamines, sympathomi-

metic amines, licorice, beer, wine, aged cheese, pickled herring, chicken liver, and chocolate.

4. Thyroid interacts with iodides and iodine-containing drugs, soy-bean preparations, brussels sprouts, cabbage, cauliflower, kale, and turnips. Cases illustrating the above interactions are in the medical literature. How significant they are remains to be seen. However, they are already with us. This, then, is the personal, internal environment that is part of the problem of describing the nature of health protection.

THE IMMEDIATE ENVIRONMENT

Merely cataloguing all the "insults" to the individual person adds little to our understanding of the nature of protection. These aggravations and manipulations of the human organism come about largely as responses to the immediate environment. This has been suggested in some of the foregoing material; at this point we can be more specific.

There was a certain subtle irony to Richard Nixon's campaign theme of "Bring Us Together" in 1968. If one could suggest several root causes of the national malaise that year, among them would no doubt be our overwhelming "togetherness." By 1970 two-thirds of our citizens occupied ten per cent of American real estate; about 160 million Americans had become "urbanized," and we anticipate the number might surpass 200 million by 1980. At the end of this century, some demographers predict, about 300 million Americans will be living in the same land areas now occupied by half that number. This is "togetherness" with a vengeance.

We are multiplying much faster than we are learning how to cope with human multiplication. Coping, of course, is another way of expressing protection. However it is expressed, the problem remains the same: the individual is undergoing extraordinary new stresses in his immediate environment—his home, his work area, his recreational and shopping areas, and even within the "envelope," so to speak, of his own family.

Stress—The interpersonal stress is without doubt the most important to consider. Health protection against such stress follows no orderly regimens of the past. This is where the tranquilizing agents have begun to play a strong role; new approaches—methodologies, philosophies, techniques—in mental health are based on interpersonal pathologies of a crowded nation; and the calendar itself is being manipulated to deliver longer weekends, vacations, sabbaticals, retreats, and other forms of physical as well as emotional and psychological release.

Sometimes, such release is not available and another kind is sought. For Americans in the prime of their lives—ages 15 through 44—suicide ranks as the fourth major cause of death. For the past decade, suicide has been among the most studied phenomena by college and university health officials. At the meetings of the American Psychological Association, this topic—the student suicide—has attracted more researchers, more papers, and larger audiences.

The attack upon one's self is the ultimate offense; protection against such an occurrence is not only complex (in terms of effective mechanisms) but may also be beyond the abilities of any of the professions now practicing in the health field. It may be that this is one reason for so much heightened activity in the past few years on other kinds of crime and crime reporting. How threatening is the immediate environment? How is it perceived? How does the individual—with or without aid—protect himself against hostilities close at hand?

Crime—A survey conducted by the President's Commission on Law Enforcement and Administration of Justice revealed that sixteen per cent of the respondents acknowledged they stay home rather than go out on certain occasions; their reason was fear of personal attack (assault, robbery, rape, or murder). A third of the blacks responded this way, against only one out of eight whites. The Crime Commission (as the group has been called) noted that the most likely victim of a major crime is a black male living in poverty in the inner city; the least likely victim is a white female living in comfort in a suburban or rural area. Readers of daily newspapers should not be surprised at these facts; they are "common knowledge." However, from crimes against the person—or from the anticipation of such crimes—comes a whole range of "illnesses" and trauma for which health professions are not yet fully equipped.

Privacy—There are other, far more subtle "crimes" persons commit against their fellows, recalling once again the challenges raised by Weinerman. For example, privacy is now a right that must be vigorously defended, or it disappears and cannot be retrieved. The private person is in all of us: even the most gregarious, outgoing exhibitionist has a private side that will not be altogether sublimated. Yet, the disintegration of privacy—and the resulting disintegration of personality and, to some extent, physiology—continues to occur. Here are two indicators not usually noticed, but pertinent nevertheless:

1. Between 1958 and 1968, the annual growth rate in sales of photographic equipment was 12.7 per cent. The 1958 sales figure was $1.2 billion; in 1968 it hit $4 billion. Included in this tabulation are not only the self-loading, self-processing, cubeflash, automatic focus and exposure

cameras for the rank amateur, but the other kind of photo equipment, the kind that may not take a picture of your face but, as an office copier, takes a "picture" of your birth certificate, marriage license, fingerprints, department-store bills, and love letters. The ways to record a man— and in endless copies—are staggering to the imagination. Yet, there is an industrial boom now in progress related to the technical ability to invade the personal "envelope" of the human.

2. Between 1958 and 1968 there was nearly a tripling in the shipments of radio and television receivers, including AM/FM clocks. In dollars, the value of shipments rose from $1.6 billion in 1958 to $4.4 billion in 1968. The general noise level of society is up, as a stroll down any apartment-house hallway will reveal. This assault upon the ears and the psyche has yet to be carefully measured and understood, so that some workable strategies for the individual—for his own personal protection—can be provided. At one time, when the bully on the beach kicked sand in your eyes, you had recourse to muscle-building and, eventually, to kicking some of that sand back. At this time the assault comes from a score of transistor radios held by otherwise quiet, unobstrusive, horizontal people. What good is a 22-inch bicep against 50 kilowatts of acid-rock? Not much good at all.

THE GENERAL ENVIRONMENT

And from the crowding, from the advances in food and drug technology, from all the strands of our highly technological civilization comes a web of general danger and distress. The threatened environment of this planet is slowly rising as the single most galvanizing issue unrelated to war. Indeed, it is widely felt that, as United States involvement in land wars overseas diminishes, the energies of its citizens will be turned to the issue that is proving to be as controversial and taxing as Vietnam: the protection of the environment.

Solid Waste Disposal—In earlier days there was much theorizing about the general environment, its possible deterioration, and what could be done to save it. Now there is much data to work with. We know, for example, that solid waste disposal in 1970 is more than a good general topic: we know that it means getting rid of 440,000 tons of rubbish every day. We know that we are producing junk and garbage at a rate rising twice as fast as our rate of population growth. We know that an average family throws out about twenty pounds of banana peels, facial tissues, no-deposit bottles, soup cans, and newspapers every day. One thing we are doing to our environment is simply loading it with garbage and rubbish. (In 1975 an estimated eight million cars will be junked. As the decade of the sixties came to a close, the rate was a little better than one million; in Chicago, one car was abandoned every seven and one half minutes; the national abandonment rate was one car per thirty minutes.) To argue the aesthetics of the matter is of little use, since the public just does not respond to this side of the problem. Yet, the protection of life and health in terms of the general environment is probably the fundamental assignment for health professionls in the last third of the twentieth century.

Hazardous Chemicals—For many years we have worried about the effect of DDT in the environment; while using it extensively during the quarter century following World War II—and extolling its ability to attack malaria and typhus, as well as agricultural pests—we have been uneasy about the fact that DDT residues have shown up in Antarctic penguins as well as Lake Michigan salmon. The concept of the "biological food chain" (algae eaten by fish eaten by birds eaten by animals eaten by man) has not really captured the interest of the public; the multiplication factor in this chain has also not been conveyed or understood. But suddenly American mothers are informed that, on the average, they produce breast milk with .2 parts per million of DDT, about four times the allowable DDT residue in cow's milk sold in grocery stores. Obviously, by the time American mothers (and fathers) wake up to the significance of this fact, it is already too late. Purging the environment—and mothers—of DDT cannot be done. The only alternative is to shut down the further production and use of DDT, and other so-called "persistent pesticides," so that more harm will not be inflicted.

Water Pollution—The biosphere—that part of the earth in which man lives—is a complex of checks and balances vaguely understood but given more and more respect as scientists and public administrators realize that it is the only biosphere we have. Yet we have viciously abused it, particularly during the past century of modern industrial development. If we continue to pour our sewage into our moving water supplies, for example, with the kind of abandon we have enjoyed thus far, it is possible (says the National Academy of Sciences) that we will simply deoxygenate those supplies by 1980.

The human organism itself is composed mostly of water, a simple fact that has had little effect upon environmental planning. As a result of erratic industrial spread, suburban sprawl, and unchecked use of agricultural chemicals, most of the nation's water is of questionable quality. About a third of the drinking water systems are below modest federal standards; yet, these same systems serve nearly half the country's population. In a biochemical sense, these Americans are "deprived" or "disadvantaged." The water they draw in from the environment is of a constantly lowered quality; the implication is a constant debasement of the human organism itself. Indeed, the threat of hepatitis, poliomyelitis, influenza, meningitis, and other water-borne diseases is now both imminent and virtually everywhere.

As if to alert us with a kind of Biblical metaphor, an American river—the Cuyahoga flowing through Cleveland to Lake Erie—caught fire in the summer of 1969. The once lovely river had become a combustible porridge of oil and industrial wastes, not unlike many other rivers, streams, and lakes. Polluted waters have become visible measuring devices of industrial advance. In mid-century the waters are choked with de-oxygenating wastes; in the last third of the century the water—what usable water may be left—is under threat of heat, thermal pollution from mammoth energy (nuclear, gas, oil) plants. As civilization moves away from fossil fuels to nuclear energy, the contamination of water from radium 226 or strontium 90 or the overheating of water spewed back into rivers from cooling systems will be the new signs of environmental abuse and danger. The thirst of man is different from—and even threatened by—the thirst of what man has made; this much we know—and that knowledge is beginning to weigh heavily upon the public in general and the health professions in particular.

Air Pollution—We are killing our babies: as simple a statement as that seems to emerge from all the facts and figures and tables and charts of the study of the general environment. Infant mortality— a cold, statistician's term—is probably the key to shaking every citizen into some comprehension of what is at stake. In June 1967, a Task Force on Environmental Health and Related Problems informed then-Secretary of Health, Education and Welfare John W. Gardner that "plans for abatement of air pollution, whether Federally developed or not, must strive for the full use of available means for reducing major air contaminants discharged from stationary sources of pollution, specifically including particulate matter, oxides of sulphur, hydrocarbons, and oxides of nitrogen." The task force called for 90 per cent reduction of these air pollutants.

On December 3, 1969, Chicago's Health Commissioner, Dr. Murray C. Brown, reported, "The death rate of tracheal bronchitis in children has been running about 50 per cent higher than was expected. These are children of crib age." Dr. Brown made his report following a seven-day period that claimed the lives of nine such infants suffering from acute tracheal bronchitis. The children died following a particularly severe period of sulphur dioxide air pollution in Chicago

(25 parts per million, a disabling or fatal level for adults). During that same period, the overall death figure was 804, or about 50 deaths more than would have been anticipated.

Dr. Brown would not say for sure whether there was a causal relationship between the sudden upturn in pollution and the jump in infant deaths ("We just don't have the scientific knowledge to determine it"), but he was ready to put all the figures into the public record. Something was happening in the general environment which was killing babies: that was a distinct possibility.

The observations of Dr. Brown in Chicago were, in microcosm, an echo of earlier rumblings in the scientific community. In the summer and fall of 1969, during the debate over the Anti-Ballistic Missile (A.B.M.) system proposed by President Nixon, a University of Pittsburgh team, headed by Ernest J. Sternglass, professor of radiation physics, released data to indicate their deep uneasiness of what we were doing in the environment that had catastrophic effects on human life.

Radiation Hazards—With the aid of a computer, the infant mortality tables of 1935–1950, the public record of atomic and hydrogen bomb tests of 1945–1962, and data on strontium 90 levels in a number of states, Sternglass came up with this kind of conclusion:

> From 1935 to 1950, the [infant mortality rate] shows a steady decline, and mathematical models allow the rate to be extended to show, on the basis of previous experience, what the infant mortality rate for any time, consistent with the immediate past, ought to be. But while elsewhere (with one exception) in the U.S. the rate continued downward as expected, in the states downwind from Alamagordo it did not. There was no change in the infant death rate in 1946—the year after the Trinity test—but by 1950 the rate in Texas, Arkansas, Louisiana, Mississippi, Alabama, Georgia, and both Carolinas deviated upward from the normal expectancy. Increases in excess infant mortality of some twenty to thirty per cent occurred some thousand to fifteen hundred miles away in Arkansas, Louisiana, and Alabama, where mortality rates were between 3 and 4.5 per hundred live births. Thus, as observed by our research group at the University of Pittsburgh, the Alamagordo blast appears to have been followed by the death, before reaching age one, of roughly one hundred children in the area downwind. No detectable increase in mortality rates relative to the computer-determined 1940–1945 baseline was observed in Florida, south of the path of the fallout cloud, or in the states to the north; and the mortality excesses become progressively less severe with increasing distance eastward, in a manner now understood to be characteristic of the activity along the path of a fallout cloud.

Sternglass and his group also plotted the relationships among radioactive fallout in selected states, the evidence of strontium 90 in milk, fetal deaths, infant mortality, such diseases as leukemia and bone cancer, and the occurrences of bomb tests around the world. The coincidences are nothing less than alarming. (A special report of the Pittsburgh studies was published in *Esquire*, September 1969.) Although there is difference within the scientific community as to the validity of such interpretations, it is clear that all these data "are trying to tell us something"—something extremely important for those who labor in the health field.

Perception of Environmental Biomedicine—As Dr. Rene Dubos has said:

> What is required is nothing less than a bold imaginative departure from orthodoxy and the creation of a new science of environmental biomedicine—a systematic science of total man in his total environment—emanating either outside the university complex, or in new academic institutions not yet committed to the orthodox fields of science. The social need for such a fresh, bold approach is acute.

As mentioned earlier in this chapter, we are accumulating a great deal of information, but it is all being screened and manipulated by personnel trained in yesterday's problems and disciplines. The problems of today and tomorrow—regarding the protection of health—are barely perceived by even the most adventurous minds. Among the many "crises" discussed by scientists, politicians, sociologists, and editorial writers, one must add this rather important "crisis of perception."

Environment as the "New Thing"

At this time in world history man is beginning to confront his own handiwork and is assessing its value. Some of it has positive value; much has negative value. These are dimly perceived, however. In 1967, Ronald Ridker produced a book entitled *Economic Costs of Air Pollution*. Ridker's conclusion: "*No* one has ventured to suggest what the magnitude of such a charge should be" mainly because the costs "require empirical information far beyond our current understanding of the problem." Early in 1969, Lord Ritchie-Calder, writing in *The Center Magazine* (published by the Fund for the Republic, Inc.) on "Polluting the Environment," observes that "The present younger generation has an unhappy awareness of such matters" as man's blundering about in atomic power, computers, space, and bioengineering. "They see the mistakes writ large," says Ritchie-Calder, adding, "But they do not have the explicit answers, either."

ENVIRONMENT AND QUALITY OF LIFE

Nevertheless, problems of the environment have captured the attention of young people in the sciences—natural, physical, and social—who want to "do something" about the "quality of life." Their uneasiness began to deepen after the generational confrontation over the war in Vietnam: young people saw they could grapple with a global issue and acquit themselves every bit as well as their elders. It is natural to see youth, therefore, pursue something as big as The Environment, Human Ecology, the Survival of the Species itself.

Aside from the technological issues involved—and they are vast—there are large, cloudy political and economic issues as well. In fact, as Garrett Hardin noted in his article, "The Tragedy of the Commons" (*Science,* 13 December, 1968), ". . . the concern here is with the important concept of a class of human problems which can be called 'no technical solution problems'. . . ." Hardin raises this interesting point in a discussion of the finite world we live in—our "commons"—and how we are desecrating it at our peril. Hardin says:

> . . . [The] tragedy of the commons reappears in probems of pollution. Here it is not a question of taking something out of the commons, but of putting something in—sewage, or chemical, radioactive, and heat wastes into water; noxious and dangerous fumes into the air; and distracting and unpleasant advertising signs into the line of sight. The calculations of utility are much the same as before. The rational man finds that his share of the cost of the wastes he discharges into the commons is less than the cost one, we are locked into a system of "fouling our own nest," so long as we behave only as independent, rational free-enterprisers.

YOUTH INVOLVEMENT IN HEALTH PROTECTION

If no technical solutions are possible, then technical solutions *coupled with* political and economic solutions might be possible. Here, young people are looking for new openings to attack the conventional wisdom everywhere, so as to preserve the environment. The beginnings are tenuous, sometimes theatrical, not always logical, occasionally effective—but all leading to a building of pressure for concern and for change. It is doubtful that the concern for the protection of life, for the health of the individual in an increasingly destructive environment, will lose its momentum among the next and succeeding generations. A data base of any consequence is lacking as we enter the 1970s; a philosophy base is absent as well. But the felt concern is evident, and that is enough of a beginning.

On September 23, 1954, Aikichi Kuboyama died. At his funeral was a large contingent of university students, who outnumbered Kuboyama's mourning family and friends. The students released the clould of white pigeons and chanted, "A-bomb never forgiven." The ceremony was orderly and simple, as was the final interment of Kuboyama's ashes on the hillside overlooking his native village of Yaizu. A decent burial for an honest fisherman is within the understanding of most of us. But the students did not just bury a man that day— they signaled the beginning of an inquiry, destined to last for the remainder of the twentieth century at least. Much of that inquiry is still only dimly understood, as Ridker, Ritchie-Calder, and others have testified. The questions rise and move out on the wind as the pigeons did that day at Yaizu. But once asked, they persist until answered. In those answers are written the ways in which man may survive in his *personal environment,* the *immediate environment,* and the *general environment.*

James Z. Appel

6

Health Care Delivery

Debate on the health of the nation has been going on with varying intensity since the close of World War II, but concern prior to 1965 was limited primarily to the financing of health care. In the early sixties there was beginning realization that merely relieving the burden of the cost for health care would not be enough. Concern was expressed in a few quarters that such measures could indeed worsen the health care picture by increasing demand far in excess of the ability of health resources to satisfy the people. Others were concerned that in spite of financial relief, the resources available would not be utilized to their capacity, limited though they might be, because of the poor distribution of manpower and facilities. Still others, looking at the health problem from a purely scientific point of view, were alarmed at the disparagement revealed in a comparison not only of international health statistics but also of those health statistics used to measure the health of Americans.

Time has justified these concerns. Medicare and Medicaid have relieved the financial impact of personal health care for the elderly and the financial barrier that has limited to some extent the procurement of health care for the indigent and medically indigent. But these two programs must accept their role among the many factors responsible for the rising costs of health care. Continued studies of our domestic health statistics reveal a great variation in the mortality,

JAMES Z. APPEL, M.D., *is a practicing physician in Lancaster, Pennsylvania. He was president of the American Medical Association in 1965–66 and has been a member of or consultant to numerous public and private health policy groups.*

morbidity, and utilization of health care among the several segments of the population: the affluent, the average, the poor, the whites, the nonwhites, the urban, the suburban, and the rural. Comparison of the concentration of health facilities and personnel in the areas of the nation which produce the most acceptable health statistics with the lack of health personnel and facilities in those areas which produce the poorest health statistics seems to justify the arguments of those who point the finger to manpower and facility distribution.

For these and other reasons, many studies have been made of practically all aspects of health care. Among the most significant recent studies are: the White House Conference on Health, November 3 and 4, 1965; the report of the National Commission on Community Health Services, 1966; a series of papers on health services research sponsored by the Health Services Research Section of the United States Public Health Service, May 1966; the report of the 1967 National Forum on Hospital and Health Affairs; the report of the National Advisory Commission on Health Manpower, November 1967; the report of the H.E.W. Secretary's Advisory Committee on Hospital Effectiveness, 1967; the National Conference on Medical Costs, June 1967; a Program Analysis Group on Delivery of Health Services for the Poor, issued by the Department of Health, Education, and Welfare, December 1967; and the report of the President's National Advisory Commission on Health Facilities, December 1968. These are only a few of the thousands of studies, discussions, and monographs stimulated by concern over health care. Much of the statistical data quoted in these reports were compiled by the National Center for Health Statistics and various health insurance groups. The passage by Congress of the Community Health Planning Act (the "Partnership for Health" Act) and the regional medical program legislation has been an effort to implement some of the recommendations found in these reports. The creation of the National Center for Health Services Research and Development is recognition that now is the time for experimenting and evaluating the economic, sociological, and organizational aspects of the health care industry and its methods of operation.

President Lyndon Johnson articulated the national health goal when he said: "Today we expect what yesterday we could not have envisioned—adequate medical care for every citizen." Good health care has become a national policy, a "right" belonging to every citizen of this nation. In order to move towards and, if at all possible, reach such a goal, an orderly and effective process of planning must be inaugurated.

The health status of the people must be critically defined. This must include the met needs as well as the unmet needs. The resources that exist in the nation must be recognized and their effectiveness evaluated. Any discussion of resources must include manpower, facilities, distribution, quality control, methods of operation and, from a broad point of view, costs. In spite of the attitude of many of our citizens that we are living in an affluent society, recognition must be given to the fact that there are limits to our manpower reservoir as well as our purse. Thus there is created some difference between needs that must be met and wants or desires that may be beyond our capabilities. It should be noted that President Johnson chose the words "adequate medical care." He apparently recognized that there are limitations on our capabilities.

Health Manpower

Manpower is usually considered of prime importance in evaluating health resources. When we think of manpower we are prone to limit our calculations to professional manpower such as physicians, nurses, and dentists. However, the health of America is delivered by a veritable industry of employees. It includes not only the above professionals but also such additional occupational categories as Ph.D. medical scientists, biophysicists, technologists, technicians, pharmacists, and administrators. Then there are the architects and engineers who design and construct the highly specialized health facilities. Designers of the organization and economy of the industry include anthropologists, sociologists, and economists. Equally important are the educators and medical research scientists who control quality through advanced education and new discoveries. Many other people are involved, or about to become involved, such as new allied health professionals, making a total of over two hundred careers that make up this huge industry of some four million people.

Today, about one of twenty of the nation's employed are involved in the health industry, the third largest in the nation. At the present rate of growth, which will be accelerated if it expects to meet the increasing demand of the people, it could become the largest by 1975. This labor force includes approximately 297,000 physicians, 96,000 dentists, 650,000 registered nurses, 300,000 licensed practical nurses, 120,000 pharmacists, and 40,000 medical laboratory technologists alone. From 1950 to 1966 the number of persons involved in the many health careers increased 90 per cent while the nation's population increased by 29 per cent.

It has been traditional when discussing manpower and manpower needs to relate them to population. The nation has about 151 practicing physicians for every 100,000 people. Progress has been made in this respect as is demonstrated when we compare this ratio to the 141 per 100,000 ratio in 1950. However, this method of determining need or satisfactory manpower supply is not acceptable in looking at the national picture, particularly as it relates to health care. It becomes more acceptable when evaluating small areas of our geography and segments of our population. The tremendous fragmentation that has developed in the medical profession by the increasing degree of specialization of its members destroys any validity of such ratios in determining sufficiency. This specialization has been undirected in any way as a response to need or demand. Rather it has proceeded more on the basis of the inclination of the medical student as to the particular specialty and by the social and economic prestige attached to specialization in general. Undoubtedly the increasing knowledge coming from the research institutions, and particularly in-depth knowledge, has not only necessitated specialization but has been attractive to those with the high intellectual caliber demanded of the prospective medical student. About 55 per cent of practicing physicians today are specialists. More to the point, in recent years only about 12 per cent of medical school graduates go into general practice.

MANPOWER DISTRIBUTION

Compounding the physician manpower problem is their distribution. The inclusion in the overall physician population of those who are primarily engaged in research and education improves the ratio of physician to population in those areas of the nation where the large medical centers are located. But more serious to the validity of the ratio as a yardstick is the concentration of practicing physicians in the metropolitan and affluent suburban sections of the nation and their scarcity in the low-income and more thinly populated areas. Even in the large population centers there are areas of great scarcity of physicians. If we compare total physician population to national population, the national ratio is one physician for every 750 people. When we develop this same ratio for each of the 50 states, we find a variation that extends from one for 280 to one for 1,400 people, according to a study by David Rutstein. In most cases those states with the least desirable ratio were the least densely populated and therefore distances interfered with availability of physicians. Even within a rural state there is variation of concentration that leaves many people without sufficient physician manpower. It is reported that in some counties in

Appalachia, especially in Kentucky and Tennessee, there is one physician for every 5,000 to 10,000 people.

Equally if not more significant is the maldistribution in our large metropolitan areas. A study by Milton Roemer in 1966 showed that in the Watts area in Los Angeles, for example, there were 106 practioners serving 251,000 people. There was a ratio of 38 to 100,000 in the southeast district and 45 to 100,000 in the south district. Seventeen of these 106 physicians classified themselves as specialists though only 5 were so certified.

The Chicago Board of Health divided that city into census tracts and reported physician to population ratios of 0.62 physicians to 1,000 persons in the poverty areas and 1.26 physicians per 1,000 persons in the non-poverty areas. In Cleveland similar findings were brought out in a study of that city by Joanne Finley in 1967. The poverty areas showed a ratio of 0.45 physicians per 1,000 population while non-poverty areas had a ratio of 1.13 physicians per 1,000 population.

These statistics are not too surprising, and are reproduced almost identically when we apply the same tests to distribution of dentists and registered nurses. The low economy of these areas, remoteness from sophisticated health facilities, poor cultural environment, and often inferior educational institutions are not attractive to physicians either as a place in which to practice medicine or to establish a home for their wives and children. Of paramount importance is the desire of the physician's wife in this regard.

PROFESSIONAL PRODUCTIVITY

Before becoming too pessimistic about these negative findings and in order to properly evaluate manpower needs, one must take a look at what has occurred to the productivity of the physician. According to the 1967 report of the National Advisory Commission on Health Manpower, from 1955 to 1965 the population of this nation increased 17 per cent while the number of active physicians increased 22 per cent. During the same time professional nurses increased 44 per cent, registered X-ray technologists increased 56 per cent and laboratory personnel increased 70 per cent. Although dentists only increased 13 per cent in the same period, dental assistants went up 32 per cent and dental hygienists 54 per cent.

These increases have had a major impact on the productivity of both professions. While the number of physicians in private practice increased 12 per cent between 1955 and 1965, "physician-directed services" increased 81 per cent and "dentist-directed services" 47 per cent.

Such services include not only the personal services of the physician or dentist but also those provided by their laboratories and staff for which the patient is billed. With a population increase of 17 per cent this means that the productivity in services rendered to the people has been markedly increased on a per capita basis. This more than explains the finding that though the number of physicians in practice increased by 8 per cent between 1959 and 1964, the total number of visits to physicians in the same period increased by only 4 per cent. If the productivity of the physician per visit was increased by the 81 per cent figure used above, then inevitably there has been a vast increase in the services rendered to the total population by the total physician manpower.

If we attempt to balance the present number of individuals who make up health manpower (taking into consideration the maldistribution and fragmentation by specialization) against the increased productivity per practicing physician and compare it with the demand by the people for services, we can only conclude that there is a manpower shortage. However, in determining our objective as to manpower needs we must remember that there is a ceiling as to what portion of the national population can be employed by the health industry without disrupting the other necessary operations of our national society. Also, just as there is a limit as to how much money can be spent efficiently on any project, so there is a limit as to the number of people who can be employed in any industry with a similar degree of efficiency. There is already evidence that in some aspects of the health industry there is inefficient overemployment. Manpower becomes wasted. But still more to the point, where there is a shortage of manpower the inefficient use of the highly skilled professionals to perform services that can be performed by lesser skilled and trained individuals who require shorter lead-time to produce is just as wasteful, one might say sinful, as pouring money down the drain.

We do need more physicians, both highly skilled specialists as well as broader trained family physicians. We do need more dentists and nurses. Our scientific advances have created needs for more Ph.D. biochemists, biophysicists, and physiologists, as well as a variety of technologists and technicians. Our existing medical, dental, and nursing schools and our broader universities must produce more trained men and women in each category. This can only be accomplished by enlarging their present capacities and by developing more schools for the health sciences.

As our educational institutions are presently designed and programmed, the lead-time required to produce such manpower is too long. Reevaluation of the present educational curriculum is essential in order to ascertain if it is necessary. Might it not be shortened in order to increase production without lowering quality of the product? Fourteen to sixteen years of education after graduation from high school is a long time to produce a surgeon.

UTILIZATION OF HEALTH PERSONNEL

Another approach to balancing manpower against need is to improve the utilization of the ancillary health personnel already trained and at work. The clinical psychologist, the pharmacist, the podiatrist and the optometrist are just a few of this group of hard-working members of the health team who could be used to relieve the short supply of the highly demanded physician. For too long professional pride and jealousy, fear of competition, and criticism of competence have restricted the cooperative arrangements that could have increased the efficient use of the skills and time of the more highly educated segments of the health professions. There is some justification for part of the fears exhibited by the medical profession with regard to the ability and at times the unwillingness of the technically trained health professional to recognize his limits. Within the medical profession itself it is just as difficult to recognize when one has a problem beyond one's ability. As a single profession, having its own self-determined codes of ethics and discipline, control does exist. There is a certain amount of skepticism, deserved or otherwise, held by the medical profession as to whether these other professions maintain equal standards.

The psychiatrist and the clinical psychologist should be able to work together to enhance each's productivity for the ultimate benefit of their patients. Mutual understanding and respect would be generated. Fear of competition and exploitation of competence would be dispelled. The same applies to the podiatrist and the orthopedist and to the ophthalmologist and the optometrist. The insistence on high standards of education by and for the limited health professionals will further these essential relationships.

Pursuing this line of thought a little further, it becomes necessary to examine critically all the functions that the highly trained physician, dentist, and nurse perform in order to determine if new and lesser trained personnel can take over some of the more repetitive routine procedures. Experimentation in the development of physician assistants is presently going on in several of our university centers, notably Duke University and the University of Colorado. For example, a study by J. Stokes in 1966 concluded that about 50 per cent of a pediatrician's office time is spent performing tasks that could equally well be performed by lesser trained individuals. Another report on the same subject goes further and estimates that 70 per cent of the pediatrician's day-to-day work could be delegated. By placing more emphasis on the use of public health nurses, two medical centers in the nation were able to reduce the number of visits of women to obstetricians by 50 per cent and to pediatricians by 75 per cent. A previous report in 1964 concluded that 20 to 30 per cent of the work performed by the general practitioner could be performed by assistants.

Physician assistants could undoubtedly perform such functions as physical screening, participation in follow-up care of the chronically ill, patient counselling, supervision of minor illnesses such as upper respiratory infections, most of the procedures involved in well baby care, guidance in family planning and, in the case of obstetrics, management of uncomplicated deliveries, as pointed out in a 1966 study by H.E.W. They would operate under the direct supervision of a physician. State laws of licensure undoubtedly would have to be altered and liability laws amended. Continued experimentation in this regard is justified by the qualified success of universities which have developed curricula for such students. Former medical corpsmen of the military services, graduate nurses from either diploma schools or baccalaureate programs, and pharmacists would make ideal candidates. However, prospective students need not be limited to these categories.

In summary, although total manpower is formidable and growing, it should not be considered optimum. Increasing demand for health services, fragmentation of the professions by specialization, maldistribution of personnel, and relative dearth of labor saving devices have already created a shortage of manpower in all fields. Moreover, the growing demand for services predicts an increasingly short supply for the future. Methods must be devised whereby education and training of manpower can be shortened, whereby labor saving devices (such as multiphasic screening and computer interpretation of ECG's and X-ray films) are developed, and better cooperation among all health professions is created.

Health Facilities

The short-term, acute-care hospitals are the keystones of the many facilities that serve as foci for the delivery of health care. Even though they provide less than one half of all hospital beds, they account for more than 85 per cent of all hospital admissions. However, the total inventory of the nation's health facilities is extensive. There are about 7,000 hospitals providing approximately 1,700,000 beds. This represents capital assets of about $28 billion. In addition there are about 12,000 skilled nursing homes with more than 600,000 beds, some 5,000 diagnostic and treatment centers, 3,000 public health centers, 4,300 medical group practice clinics, and many thousands of physicians' and dentists' offices.

These facilities are the product of both private enterprise and government funding. An example is the Hill-Burton program which has assisted 3,700 communities in the building of hospitals and nursing homes providing more than 400,000 beds. In addition during the twenty years before 1969 it assisted in financing the construction of 1,200 public health centers, over 900 diagnostic and treatment centers, and over 400 rehabilitation centers. Since Hill-Burton grants require two dollars of state or local funds for each dollar of federal money, past federal grants of $3.1 billion have generated $10 billion of capital investment in health facilities since 1946.

As originally enacted this federal legislation was aimed at the improvement of health facilities in rural and low per capita income areas. Thanks as well to the initiative and concern of rural America for the health of its people, physical distance from available hospital care is not a major barrier for rural residents. Only two per cent of the population live more than 25 miles from a hospital facility of 25 beds or more. Furthermore only one per cent must travel more than 50 miles to obtain services of such a facility. An hour's drive for such routine purposes as shopping and entertainment is commonplace. With the exception of extreme emergencies, such distribution of health facilities should not create difficulties in the procurement of hospital care.

In the urban areas everyone lives within ten miles of a hospital. On the surface this does not appear unreasonable. For in-patient care it probably does not create much deterrence. But for the poor, without personal transportation, dependent upon mass transportation and repeated out-patient services for their health care, an eight to ten mile trip by bus requiring one hour and costing 68 cents one way, as it does in the Watts area of Los Angeles, presents a formidable problem. The financial burden is increased when this time and cost are compounded by the long wait at the out-patient department of the hospital for the employed worker, by loss of wages and cost of a baby sitter for a mother.

As we look at these urban hospitals there is apparent one problem which Hill-Burton in its original concept failed to rectify. Hospitals were built with fairly good per capita bed capacity for the urban community which they served. However, because of age as well as advances in health care they are, or are rapidly becoming, obsolete. In 1968 it was estimated, as reported by the National Advisory Commission on Health Facilities, that it would require $10 billion to correct present obsolescence and another $10 billion would be needed to overcome the obsolescence that would develop in the ensuing ten years. Congress has taken steps to correct this situation and some grants have been authorized. But it is a big problem and its solution will take time.

HOSPITAL AS SUBSTITUTE FOR PRIMARY PHYSICIAN

It has been pointed out that there is a shortage of physicians, particularly in those sections, urban or rural, which are not attractive to practitioners. Thus many people by necessity or choice utilize the community hospitals' emergency and out-patient departments in lieu of a primary physician. As a rule, community hospitals are primarily concerned with and organized for in-patient care and for the rendition of a large array of laboratory diagnostic services. Their emergency departments are organized and equipped to take care of true emergencies. As to the routine care of ambulatory patients, they offer little in the way of continuity.

The out-patient departments in most community hospitals were developed almost as an afterthought to take care of "charity" cases, not as a substitute for the primary physician. In hospitals these departments have long been financially a debit item. They have been given low priority by both administration and staff. This certainly is not as it should be, but it is a fact of life. Thus patients who use these out-patient facilities (and their numbers are increasing) have justifiable complaints as to environment, long waiting, and impersonal and all too often poor service.

The in-patient facilities of most of the community hospitals built more than four or five years ago were designed with little thought given to planning for efficient operation and practically no consideration to ease of remodeling. They were designed as segregated units, department by department, rather than a coordinated whole. The purpose of the hospital was to be a facility equipped and staffed to diagnose and treat the acutely ill. The fact that the convalescent patient, the chronically ill patient, and the patient in need of rehabilitation therapy do not need the type of facility designed for the acutely ill with its high manpower requirement was apparently given little thought. Patients should be treated in the type of facility required to meet the medical needs of the patient and nothing more. Therefore facility designing should be directed to accomplish this, with consequential manpower saving.

As advances occurred one on top of the other in medical sciences and as these required special facilities, it was soon found that the traditional designing of the "memorial-type" hospital barred any effort to remodel for these new functions, at least in any practical way. Thus provision must be made for flexibility incorporated in the original design that will permit remodeling as needed.

TYPES OF FACILITIES

Hospitals are not the only facilities of the health care industry. The chronically ill are cared for in institutions such as nursing homes, convalescent homes, custodial homes, homes for the aged, and more recently, extended care facilities. Prior to the passage of Medicare and Medicaid these facilities were low in number and poor in quality. However, there has been a boom in the construction and staffing of such institutions, which are presently giving good service in well designed and equipped buildings and thus to some extent relieve the overcrowding of the acute care hospitals. Estimates have been made that at times 30 per cent of the patients in a given acute care hospital do not need the services there available but will do just as well if not better in an institution designed for extended care or rehabilitation, with a consequent saving of manpower.

Additional types of facilities are beginning to play prominent roles in health care: group clinics, either organized by physicians of a variety of specialties or by a third party such as the Kaiser Industries or a labor union; partnerships, which are usually several physicians of the same specialty; diagnostic and treatment centers; and more recently neighborhood health centers. Some of these facilities are associated administratively or geographically with a hospital or medical center. Others are autonomous facilities remotely located from a center.

Finally, there are the governmental (national and state) institutions. These include military installations, veterans, hospitals, public health facilities for special categories of people such as the Indians, and the special category disease institutions such as the National Institutes of Health (N.I.H.) and the narcotics hospitals. At the state level there are institutions particularly directed to the care of chronic diseases such as mental disease, tuberculosis and other chronic respiratory diseases.

Types of Practice Organization—Perhaps we might diverge from this train of thought for a moment to discuss briefly the debate concerning solo practice, specialty group practice or partnerships, and multidisciplinary group clinics. Each of these methods can and does provide good quality medical care. Each has disadvantages for both consumer and provider.

There can be developed a more personal and intimate relationship between patient and physician in the solo practice of medicine than in either of the other two methods. The inclusion of a family type physician, be he general practitioner or general internist, on the staff of a group clinic with the formal responsibility for the care of specific patients or families tends to overcome this apparent weakness of the clinic arrangement.

It is probably true that the consumer selecting a solo practitioner as his private physician has more freedon of choice than if he selects or enrolls in a group practice clinic. In the latter case, when specialty care is indicated, he is captured by the clinic organization. However, it is true that most patients are not in a position to make valid judgments as to the relative expertise of the specialists in their community. They must rely largely upon the advice and guidance of their primary physician. It can not be said that the latter's referral selection is entirely unbiased. Many factors other than qualifications affect his decision in making referrals. The captivity of a clinic patient is somewhat mitigated by the selection process used in the recruitment of physicians by a clinic staff.

Fee-for-service is the prevailing method of payment for services rendered by solo physicians. While the same system can and often is used in clinic practice and partnerships, the ultimate result in the form of income to the physician who renders the service is usually a form of salary plus payment. Fee-for-service acts as an incentive for better performance to some people in or out of medicine. It also identifies the cost of each service the patient is purchasing. On the other hand it does not insure a definite income for the provider, thus making it somewhat difficult for him to budget his personal living costs. Some physicians need this incentive for better performance; others do not, and perform better because they can completely divorce their personal economic concerns from their professional problems. The incentives of fee-for-service can become so strong as to tempt physicians, to say the least, to overtreatment.

In solo practice the physician theoretically has complete control over his working conditions. He is not regimented to definite hours of work, fixed vacations, and methods of practice. However, if he is truly conscientious he will not exercise this control to the detriment of his patient. In fact many become the slaves of their practice. In partnerships and clinics hours of work are regulated. This provides definite hours during which the physician is off-duty when he can relax, study, and enjoy his family. Predetermined vacations are insured. Unfortunately too many group clinics do not provide for home coverage and 24-hour service seven days each week. This can be taken care of but requires more manpower.

With the larger organization of the two forms of group practice more types of medical and ancillary services can be made available to the ambulatory patient under one roof than is possible for the solo practitioner. The clinic thus takes on more and more the character of the department store or shopping center. Just as these two forms of merchandising are attractive to the consumer by their conveniences, so the clinic provides a convenience that the soloist or single disciplinary group can not match. This centralization of specialists and services in one organization can lessen the demand for unnecessary in-hospital service.

At present there is no valid method of evaluating the quality of the services rendered in the home of the patient or the office of the practitioner who operates solo or in a small partnership. Using the same techniques of peer review practiced in hospitals (discussed elsewhere in this chapter), group clinics can exercise effective evaluation of the quality of their service. So long as the solo practice of medicine and small partnership arrangements continue, research is indicated to develop some method of evaluation of their quality.

Large group clinics, especially those associated with a hospital, have been able to demonstrate better cost control to the benefit of the consumer than has been accomplished by solo practitioners and single disciplinary partnerships. But cost control in large group clinics can itself get out of hand and unduly restrict the professional freedom of the medical staff. Services which demonstrate a marginal cost effectiveness, but which are needed by the consumers, may be discontinued or severely limited by the administration of the clinic, unless professional needs of the consumer are permitted to exercise some effect upon such administrative decision making.

Continuity of care can be practiced in all three methods. It is probably simpler to perform in the multidisciplinary clinic than in the other two forms of practice, providing the clinic does include in its organization some form of primary physician assigned or accepted by the patient as his personal physician. Without this physician on the clinic staff, continuity of care suffers. In the solo practice and general practitioner partnership, continuity of care becomes automatic with the return of the patient after specialty consultation or service. Follow-up by the primary physician during the period of specialty treatment does become more difficult and is often neglected.

From the above it appears that the traditional form of solo practice in medicine is slowly dying out just as the old fashioned family doctor. While some people, perhaps most people, yearn for the close personal relationship with their physician that only the soloist can provide, they do not place as high a priority on this aspect of their medical care. The convenience, the efficiency, and the breadth of services available in the multidisciplinary clinic organization outweigh the personal touch. This not only applies to the developing attitudes of the consumer but also those of the physician provider. The clinic can provide all the desirable points of the soloist if it so desires. It will, if the patients demand it. However, the format of the clinic, its size, and its services will be dependent upon its location, the size of the community, and its relationship with medical centers and in-patient facilities. It may consist of two or three physicians and several ancillary personnel, such as a satellite of a more extensive establishment. It may be larger as in the case of neighborhood health centers now being developed in the ghettos of the metropolitan centers. It will pattern itself to the needs of the people it serves.

Education and Research

Backing up the providers of health services, both manpower and facilities, are the extensive systems of education and research. With the tremendous impetus given to research by the largest of private foundations, the competition of phamaceutical manufactures, and the appropriations by the federal government, especially through the National Institutes of Health, medical research has grown by leaps and bounds. The United States has supported medical research to the tune of $2.5 billion annually. This amounts to ten per cent of the total dollars spent for all research and development. With this kind of money there have been established not only the finest research institutions anywhere but also the greatest quantity of research as well as some of the most productive in the world.

Not all but most research efforts have become centered in our medical education institutions. It is the objective of the educator to communicate to the student both established knowledge and the gaps of knowledge. Incumbent upon this objective is the compulsion to fill the gaps. This can only be accomplished by research. Therefore, by providing incentives for research, there are attached to the profession of medical education many brilliant scientists, driven by an innate curiosity, who not only bring to the students the most recent advances in medical knowledge but also infect them with similar curiosity. But it also brings to the teaching specialty of medicine some physicians and medical scientists who have no propensity or desire for teaching. The teaching function has suffered from a lack of comparable financial support, creating an imbalance between research and teaching. Although massive support for research has been a decided educational asset to medical schools, additional support of teaching is both needed and warranted. The medical schools of this country provide an undergraduate education second to none. Through the combined efforts of the American Association of Medical Colleges, the American Medical Association, and the respective specialty associations, a post graduate system has been developed for the higher education necessary to insure that specialty care will be delivered by qualified physicians. The year 1970 saw the last type of physician, the family physician, included in the designation of specialist.

Admission standards for undergraduate medical schools are high; therefore competition for admission is keen. Undoubtedly many young men and women who aspire to a medical career are discouraged in the premedical years and turn to other pursuits. But the attraction to medicine as a career is so great that qualified applicants amount to two or three times the number that can be admitted annually. How many potentially good physicians are lost by both the high standards for admission and the limited capacity of medical schools is anybody's guess.

Medical educators are doing something about the limited capacity. In the three years before 1970, thirteen new medical schools were being developed. Many existing medical schools are enlarging their classes. As direct financial aid increases, medical schools are able to initiate recruitment drives to attract qualified young people from minority groups and the less affluent.

If the drive to enlarge our output of physicians by increasing the size and number of medical schools is to succeed, it will be a long time before much effect is noted. Under the present system it takes most students twelve to sixteen years beyond high school before they are ready to practice. The brighter students might shave these figures by two years if they are admitted to medical school after only two years of premedical education. While there has been discussion of reevaluating curriculum to shorten this educational process, there has been little implementation. Some telescoping of premedical and undergraduate medical education has occurred. The development of the trimester system and other reorganization of the academic year have speeded learning in a few instances. There are experiments breaking down the rigidity of departmental curriculum through multidepartmental curriculi, but these do little to shorten the lead time now required to produce a physician.

Pattern of Health Care Delivery

Recently there have been repeated accusations that the health care system of this nation is a "no system." It is either unorganized or poorly organized. There exists no coordination and no cooperation among various segments. If by "no system" is meant that there is no rigid single pathway to obtain health care, no control centrally directed to the placement of health personnel and facilities, and no determination by some authority as to the extent of health services which will be available in any given location or institution, this accusation may have some validity. Actually an organized system of delivery of health care has developed in a pragmatic manner and to a large extent by voluntary decision making of providers as well as consumers. It is based on a reputation for excellent performance which determines "the lines of drift" within geographic areas.

The portals of entry to the system are physicians' private offices, including partnership facilities, professional or private clinics, a variety of health centers, and out-patient departments of hospitals. Voluntary health agencies play a large role not only in diagnosis and treatment but also in case finding. This latter role is also carried out by public health nurses, social workers, and pharmacists. There have been estimates that as much as 80 per cent of the illnesses seen at the portal of entry can be satisfactorily treated there. To assist in arriving at a diagnosis, the personnel of the portal of entry utilize either their own radiological and laboratory facilities or refer their patients to more sophisticated diagnostic centers, hospitals, or commercial laboratories. While treatment in the home occurs much less than formerly, it still does occur especially in the more affluent areas. When the diagnosis requires more extensive treatment, each portal of entry has some nearby community general hospital to which the patient may be referred. When the provider of services or in many cases the consumer deems the services available in the community hospital are not of sufficient sophistication to meet the needs of the patient, there are medical centers within reasonable distance. In other words, the "line of drift" has been established from the simple to the more complex problems of diagnosis and treatment. This has functioned smoothly, especially when the extent of overdemand is taken into consideration.

Effectiveness of Health Care

In spite of all the expert manpower, all the facilities available, and the vast investment of this nation's wealth, estimated to be $60 billion in 1969, many health needs are not being met. While one can not be completely satisfied with the present accepted yardsticks for comparing a nation's health status and thus in turn for measuring quality of care, until we can agree on a better one we must depend on vital statistics. In these respects we do not compare well with many other nations. Our rates of infant and maternal morbidity and mortality when compared with those of other nations are not statistics in which we should take great pride, even though their validity is subject to some challenge because of the differences in basic definitions.

Approaching self-evaluation from a different angle, we can break down our own health statistics into such categories as age, geography, social and economic condition of life. When we do this we uncover some very interesting facts.

Applying mortality rates as a measurement of quality of health care within the total population of the United States proves to be a little difficult if we are interested in rates by income level. However certain cities have developed vital statistics by census tracts of poverty and nonpoverty "areas." In Chicago the infant mortality, neonatal mortality, and postneonatal rates were appreciably higher in the poverty areas than in the nonpoverty areas. In New York City mortality rates for cardio-vascular renal diseases, pneumonia-influenza, and accidents were definitely higher in the lower class areas than in middle class areas of the city. In the lower class area, infant mortality per thousand was approximately twice that in the middle class area.

If we equate the nonwhite population with low income we can apply those comparative statistics available for white and nonwhite segments of the total population to poverty and nonpoverty population groups. There have been significant increases in life expentancy for the newborn among both nonwhites and whites, but there still remains a 10 per cent differential in favor of the white population. Likewise, although death rates have been falling over the past 60 years, the nonwhites at a greater rate than the whites, there is still a 36 per cent differential between the groups, with the higher rate depicting the nonwhite. The nonwhite maternal mortality is approximately four times that among white mothers. The same is true for neonatal and postneonatal mortality rates. Nonwhites have a mortality rate twice that of whites for such diseases as tuberculosis, influenza-pneumonia, cerebral vascular diseases and homicide. Likewise, a higher mortality rate for cancer of the cervix is found among nonwhites.

Looking at morbidity, there is more chronic illness resulting in limitation of activity such as heart disease, arthritis and rheumatism, and orthopedic impairments among the lower income groups than the higher ones. Frequency of repeated hospitalization and length of stay in the hospital are greater in the income group under $2,000 per year. Disability days from all types of illnesses and injuries are greater in the lower income members of our society. Numerous studies indicate that the lowest income class runs a significantly higher mental health risk than the highest income class.

Another way of looking at the problem is the utilization of physicians and dentists. There occur about 900 million to a billion physician visits and about 250 million dental visits each year. However, about fifteen per cent of the people have not seen a physician in the past two years and eighteen per cent have never seen a dentist. One factor that may contribute to these statistics is undoubtedly the unequal distribution of physicians and dentists. However, the higher incidence of less frequent physician or dentist visits occurs among persons of low economic status.

From the above it might justifiably be concluded that lack of finances is a deterrent to securing needed health services. There are other factors. When the educational status of the head of the family is tabulated with family income, it is found that where the family income was less than $4,000.00 only 43 per cent of the persons were members of families in which the head of the family had completed more than eight years of schooling. In families with incomes of $4,000 to $6,999 this percentage increases to 70 per cent, and when the income amounted to $7,000, over 83 per cent of the heads of the family had more than eight years of schooling. Undoubtedly knowledge of need for physician and dental care is a factor involved in utilization.

Considering another category, place of residence, the same relations exist as to incidence of chronic diseases and extent of restricted activity and bed disability when comparing rural and urban income groups. The relationship of physician visits by income grouping is also the same in these population areas. However, there does appear to be less utilization of physician visits in the rural areas by income groups than in the urban areas, with little difference occurring in health status as measured by incidence of chronic disease and disability arising therefrom.

Recognizing the limited reliability of the above criteria as determinants of health status, it is still clear that the people who receive the least health care and need it the most are the lower income groups, both urban and rural. In searching for explanations for this picture certain barriers stand out quite clearly. Certainly shortages of manpower in both numbers and distribution create difficulties for all people but more so for the poor. It forces them to seek care in the out-patient facilities of hospitals if they are within reach. Care rendered in the traditional type out-patient department is not always of the highest type, its method of delivery is often inadequate, discriminatory and frustrating, and poor distribution of such facilities creates difficulties for the very group that applies to them.

The fragmentation of the medical profession into specialties and the resulting fragmentation within clinic and out-patient departments have not only further created manpower shortages, especially at the portal of entry, but they have also made it difficult for the less educated to determine what type of service is needed. Studies have indicated that "blue collar" workers are less informed about illness, more skeptical about the value of prevention and early treatment of an illness, and thus will seek treatment at a relatively late stage of a disease, as contrasted with the attitudes and behavior of the "white collar" worker. Undoubtedly the cost of health care is a deterrent to seeking it and has greater impact on the lower income, less well educated groups. While it may be difficult to prove statistically, racial discrimination must be considered as a factor explaining the differences of the health care received by the white and nonwhite populations at all levels of family income.

Essentials of Health Care

In effecting changes in the delivery of health services by any means certain criteria or standards must be observed. The entry into the health industry by the consumer must be accessible and acceptable. The providers must be well qualified. There must be sufficient manpower in all categories, distributed geographically so that no area of the nation is without it. Efficient use of the skills of health personnel must be insured so that their productivity is maximum and their time is not wasted in tasks which their training does not justify. Programs must be available to keep personnel abreast of the new knowledge constantly flowing from ongoing research. Incentive must be given the members of the health team to participate in such continuing education programs. Quality control of services delivered must be established through formally organized and objectively administered peer review.

In view of the importance of developing a satisfactory personal relationship between provider and consumer, free choice should be the right of both provider (physician) and consumer (patient). Health services should be available to the people at a price they can afford. On the other hand the providers of service are entitled to recompense commensurate with their skill and the investment required of them to obtain such skill and to administer the service they render.

Facilities of various types should be developed in an orderly manner so that geographically they are readily available to the people they are designed to serve. They should be equipped and staffed to avoid unnecessary duplication of services and the omission of needed services. The architectural design of health facilities should aim at efficient operation with the optimum cost-effectiveness that can be accomplished with present knowledge. Flexibility of design should be built in so that economical alterations to meet new developments in medical science and methods of administration and operation are practical. Since the cost of manpower constitutes about 70 per cent of the total cost of operating a health facility, and since the extent of personal service needed by a patient is dependent upon the type of illness he has, as well as the stage of treatment necessary, health facilities should be planned to take advantage of the varying manpower requirements of a patient. A patient should be assigned only to the type of facility designed to meet his medical needs—with consequent manpower savings.

The fragmentation of the health professions into many specialties is in one sense an artificial, arbitrarily man-made method whereby the professionals are able to master the extensive medical knowledge amassed over the years. However the patient, ill or healthy, is a whole person. The person is made up of many systems and subsystems that by and large correspond to the specialties and subspecialties. But in the person these systems and subsystems act and interact as a coordinated whole in the presence of good health. The wear and tear of life exposes this whole person to successive attacks by agents which primarily affect individual systems but through this interaction exert some distortion of other systems. Some of these effects are long lived, some are short lived. Nevertheless the rigidity of specialization can not be permitted to interfere with the concept of the whole person.

In addition to the above, there is another vertical fragmentation of the health service industry. This is the specialization of facilities from the least sophisticated one, the portal of entry (be it physician's office, neighborhood health center, or hospital out-patient department), to the most highly technical and sophisticated university medical center.

Most illnesses can be completely handled in the portal of entry. But about twenty per cent of the illnesses must move up varying steps of the ladder to a level of diagnosis and/or treatment. To avoid unnecessary duplication there must be communication from one step to another up the ladder and as the patient returns to health similar communications down.

To combat the pitfalls of these two forms of fragmentation, there has been evolved the concept of continuity of care. Continuity was simple when virtually all health care was delivered by the family physician. Today it includes not only communication of findings in the form of adequate records but also efficient referral mechanisms, ease of transportation from home to facility and from facility to facility and, in this day of a very mobile population, transference of personal health records from one geographical area to another.

Improving Health Care

It becomes obvious that the first efforts to improve American health should be directed toward those areas which presently exhibit the lowest health status and receive the poorest health service—the lower income groups both urban and rural. This does not mean that the rest of the population is to be ignored. New techniques which are developed in one group will spill over to others, so everyone benefits.

It becomes clear that there needs to be instituted some type of planning and perhaps some control that will produce more effective health care. However, the United States is a large, diverse nation, geographically, sociologically, and economically. In spite of our extensive public and private educational systems, there are great variations in the knowledge level of our people. These differences exist not only in the nation but also within each state, region, and locality.

LOCAL HEALTH PLANNING

Thus no single well organized system for the delivery of health services will be satisfactory for every community or region of the nation. Each must devise a system which best meets its needs. To do this each must examine itself and define its own goals. Resources must be determined and related to health needs. Deficiencies must be corrected either by the resources within the community or by relationships with facilities in other jurisdictions so that the seldom used and more sophisticated health measures present in other areas become available to the people in need. Unnecessary reduplication within a community must be avoided.

To accomplish this requires formal planning by each community for comprehensive health care for all. Planning at one political level should relate to planning in adjacent areas as well as with the planning of both the larger and smaller areas of the nation. Planning areas need not be determined by legal boundaries such as city, county, or state. Rather their boundaries and jurisdiction should coincide with the already defined health catchment areas, thus corresponding to the "lines of drift" already established.

To secure the cooperation required for successful planning and implementation, all health agencies must be induced to believe and participate in the planning process. All levels of consumers of health services must be active in the program. Government has a responsibility in the delivery of health care both as a provider to some selected categories (such as the military and the Indians) and as a fiscal agent. Therefore government at all levels must constitute the third leg of the planning stool.

PLANNING ELEMENTS

If voluntary cooperation cannot be satisfactorily achieved, it may be necessary to develop a "stick" to enforce adherence to accepted programs. Since government is a significant provider of funds for construction and operations, government should approve applications for financial aid only after it has reviewed the recommendations of the planning group for the area in which the proposed project is located.

Individual As Focus—In portraying existing facilities and services and filling the gaps, planners tend to develop elaborate diagrams and tables of organization. In doing so they too often place in the heart of the diagram the medical center with routes of movement from the periphery. Actually the center, the focal point, should be the individual person in need of service. In its process of reorganizing health services the planning body should start with this individual. It will thereby first develop adequate portals of entry which are best suited for the individual, the social complexion of the community, the available manpower, and the community pocketbook.

Distribution of Services—Incentives must be developed for better distribution of health professionals either in private offices, neighborhood health centers, improved hospital out-patient departments, group clinics, or mobile diagnostic and treatment teams. Contractural pathways from the portals of entry to the community hospital or specialty diagnostic center and from there to the medical center must be established so that medical records can be transferred and in some cases transportation of the patient provided. There should also be effectual relationships among the staffs of the several facilities. Such measures will provide better continuity of care for the patient and educational experience for the professional staffs.

Health Education—It has been demonstrated that easy access to services and relief from financial barriers do not necessarily lead to optimum utilization. Through ignorance, apathy or fear, many people do not seek the care they need. Therefore we must have better provision for health education and case finding. Public health nurses, school nurses, social workers, public assistance case workers and aides recruited from the area served and trained within the portal of entry can do a good job on a person-to-person basis. Health education and case finding should not stop at diagnosis, treatment, and rehabilitation but should also be concerned with preventive medicine.

Optimum Utilization—On the other hand there must be better methods of controlling misusage and overutilization of facilities and services. The tremendous advances in medical technology, "miracle" drugs, and "artificial" devices, dramatized by the news media, have produced in the public mind expectations far beyond the means of fulfilling them. The public has been oversold on the capabilities of health care. Dr. David Rutstein pointed out that "public interest, knowledge and support are all necessary to the progress of medicine. With carefully designed public education programs under professional leadership, the current unreasonable public expectation and confused demands could be guided into productive channels."

The active phase of controlling overutilization can be carried out only by the medical and dental professions. Only they can pass valid judgment upon whether a patient needs treatment, or where, or for how long. For many years the medical profession through a variety of auditing techniques has experimented with and exercised this responsibility. Medical audits, tissue committees, and more recently utilization review committees have long been in operation. Sufficient data have been obtained to evaluate their effectiveness. By reviewing the deliberations of these peer review bodies working in comparable facilities, one can develop standards and criteria of good care and utilization.

The primary purpose of peer review is quality control and not action to conserve money or bed occupancy. While the physician is and should be interested in the patient's pocketbook, he is firmly of the opinion that a healthy life has no price tag and that cost should not be a major factor in determining quality care. When a third party accepts the responsibility of financing health care it must accept the responsibility of refraining from causing a deterioration of quality care by insufficient financing.

Overtreatment and overdiagnosis are often just as harmful and have the same adverse effect on quality as undertreatment and underdiagnosis. Thus utilization, as presently considered, does become a criterion for evaluating quality care. It is an integral part of any "peer review" mechanism.

The newer programs for financing health care, including federal and private insurance, have helped many people, but they have not solved the poor health status of the lower economic group. They have exerted three side effects: they have pinpointed the real cost of health care for all to see; they have generated a demand for health services that present facilities and manpower can not satisfy; and they have increased the cost of health care through this overdemand.

Management Efficiency—Unlike the tangible product of the manufacturing industry, the product of the health industry is a personal service. Thus the conventional use of labor-saving devices, assembly line production, and automation as cost control mechanisms have had less effective application. Until recent years there has been little effect and less success in developing such measures in the health industry. The application of systems engineering to organization and design, the development of safe and economical disposable equipment, and the designing and programming of computers specifically to meet health services' needs are all in their infancy. These infants are growing rapidly. They are beginning to have an impact on controlling the acceleration of costs.

Hope for containing health costs must rest on adequate manpower and facilities, efficient organization and operation, and reduction of overutilization. The simple increase in the number of physicians, dentists and nurses, and the building of more medical, dental and nursing schools, hospitals and other health facilities will not do the job completely and may prove impractical. Increasing productivity becomes the vital goal to which this nation must direct its efforts.

Broad Participation—In order to accomplish all these improvements, the traditional concepts as to what and who constitute the health team must be considerably broadened. Physicians, dentists, nurses, pharmacists and all their assistants, aides, technologists, technicians, and administrators can not possibly do the job. The sociologists, economists, anthropologists, architects, construction and systems engineers, Ph.D. scientists, and the statistician and computer scientists and hosts of others all constitute the health team. No one profession can be "The

Leader." Each group has its own expertise and must lead in its own field. Each group must respect the other and at the same time exhibit dedicated cooperation with the others to constitute a whole.

Nor can the consumer be ignored or neglected. He too has a significant role to play and responsibility to exercise. There is a trend today that in all planning and operational boards, there shall be a majority representative of consumers. There is serious question to the validity of this trend. Health care is a highly technical enterprise. It requires direction by those well versed in the highly complicated technological and professional aspects of the industry. When human desires as expressed by consumers supersede needs and capabilities, unfamiliarity with the problems involved may well create frustrations and inefficiencies. Quantity may become so important as to destroy quality. The consumers' desires, ideas, opinions, and reactions must be voiced at high levels in the industry. The industry exists for the consumer and he should be listened to attentively and heeded. Well selected, dedicated, and knowledgeable consumers will make an effective contribution. Poorly selected consumers with emphasis on numbers will provide only disorganization and confusion.

Evaluation—Just as auditing is important in safeguarding quality of care, so is continuing evaluation essential to any planning program. It must be considered just as important as determining resources and identifying needs.

In planning, evaluation concerns itself with the continuing examination of both the planning process itself and the effectiveness of the delivery system. Inevitably, well planned programs will show flaws after implementation, which should quickly be identified and corrected. Then too it is almost axiomatic that correction of one problem generates others.

Because the process of community planning is a new approach to delivery of health service and care, innovative techniques and organizational structures must be applied. Solutions will vary from one community to another. The experiences of one planning agency should be available to other agencies. It would be well to have a central repository for such information and from which it can be disseminated throughout the nation.

The Congress of the United States has developed the National Center for Health Services Research and Development. This could well become the N.I.H. for the socioeconomic side of health care. Its purpose is to promote research and experiment in methods of improving the delivery and financing of health services. It might well function as this center of information.

Conclusion

The enemies of good health are not just bacteria, viruses, and trauma; health is related to the conditions under which people live. Their homes, their food, their work, their play, the air they breathe, the water they drink, the cleanliness of their environment, their economy, their education, and the kind of life they lead—all contribute to both good and bad health. Any attempts to improve the health of this nation must include efforts to improve these many environmental factors. Thus, planning efforts for health care must relate to all other planning efforts of the community, area, or region.

It is doubtful that we will reach our goal of optimum health care for everyone in the United States, but this must be the ideal toward which we are constantly striving. It will cost money, lots of money. It will cost great dedication and self-restraint. It will require the acceptance by each person of a self-responsibility for maintenance of health, good living, and respect for the other fellow. We as a people must decide how strongly we desire this optimum. We must set priorities for our national life. We must decide if we desire to divert a sufficient portion of the national economy to make this health goal possible and refrain from the type of life that might be pleasurable but at the same time is harmful to health.

In doing these things, let us be guided by a prayer offered by the eminent clergyman, Dr. Reinhold Niebuhr:

> O God, give us the courage to accept with serenity the things we cannot change. Give us the courage to change the things that should be changed. And give us the wisdom to distinguish the one from the other.

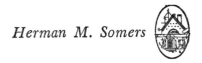

Herman M. Somers

7

Health Care Cost

Health care costs represent more than financial questions. Widespread anxiety and considerable criticism are increasingly articulated about the sharp increases in price and the fact that health services are consuming a steadily larger share of our incomes. It is true that the phenomenon has reached proportions to make it a serious national problem. Cost experience is not, however, an independent or isolated happening. It informs us not only of how much we are paying. If viewed analytically, cost data can serve as essential signals and indicators respecting virtually all issues in the organization, financing, and delivery of health care.

When prices evidence highly unusual or inconsistent patterns, they are usually signs of maladjustment between supply and demand. Such maladjustment may merely represent a temporary transitional period toward a changed level of stability, or it may bespeak more profound structural inadequacies which may not be self-correcting. Unit price and other cost data will not in themselves reveal all the complex causes, and surely not the solutions. But if their signals are properly observed, they can tell us when and where there is trouble that needs attending.

Our recent history has, in fact, moved in accordance with such a pattern. Public concern was first expressed in reaction to the stagger-

HERMAN M. SOMERS *is professor of politics and public affairs at Princeton University. Author of widely used books on medical care, he has been consultant to private and public organizations, including the health task forces of Presidents Kennedy and Johnson and the H.E.W. task force on Medicaid. Dr. Somers wrote for The American Assembly in the 1954 program on federal government services.*

ing inflation of prices, an inflation unmatched in intensity and duration. It was this experience, and its attendant resentments, that focused an unprecedented bright spotlight on the health care industry. Once the glare began to penetrate the many recesses of this complex field, it appeared to reveal an array of alleged difficulties: a delivery system (or "non-system" as it is often called) fraught with inefficiency, obsolete arrangements, inequities, and waste—all increasingly criticized by the professionals as well as laymen, but apparently intractable to quick or obvious reform.

Indicative of the heights of public policy to which the broad issue has advanced, on July 10, 1969, the President of the United States forecast over national television a "massive crisis" in health care within the next two or three years unless prompt action were taken. The occasion was his receipt of a White House report on health care needs from the Secretary of Health, Education and Welfare and the Assistant Secretary for Health and Scientific Affairs, which stated, "This nation is faced with a breakdown in the delivery of health care unless immediate concerted action is taken by Government and the private sector."

The two phenomena—high costs and a disjointed or inadequate delivery system—nurture one another. The now common awareness of the relationship has resulted in a considerably higher level of sophistication in health care cost discussions than was prevalent only a few years ago. It has become clear to most critics that the problem will not be met successfully by dependence on arbitrary price fixing, price ceilings, or any instruments exclusively directed to dollar controls, although such devices are not to be disregarded. Their concern has been drawn increasingly to the delivery system, its productivity, its adequacy, and effectiveness. This has enhanced quality consciousness, sensitivity to the wide variations in value of particular services—a problem gradually being shorn of the veil of professional mystique.

In short, it was the highly visible, widely felt, cost pressure, initially generating only price complaints, that now more than any single stimulus has made public issues of virtually all elements in the organization and financing of health care. All these elements, and the degree of their effectiveness, find expression in the costs of service. The movement is a rational response to the inevitable question: What are we getting for our money?

National Expenditure for Health Care

Total expenditures for health care in the fiscal year ending June 30, 1969, continued their long rapid increase and reached $60.3

billion. Total outlays rose $6.4 billion, or 12 per cent, in one year. Per capita expenditures, which reached $294, were almost four times as large as in fiscal year 1949–50, averaging an increase of 7.2 per cent each year.

Health expenditures have for a long time been rising faster than the nation's total output of goods and services. (See Table I.) In fiscal year 1949–50, health outlays were 4.6 per cent of gross national product; by 1968–69 they were 6.7 per cent. In 19 years health care enlarged its share of GNP by 46 per cent, in 40 years by 86 per cent. It must be remembered that the American economy has been expanding vigorously, eightfold in the last 40 years. Even if health expenditures had remained in a constant relationship to the rest of the economy, they would have experienced a substantial steady growth. But the rate at which health outlays have been outpacing GNP has been accelerating. Expenditures may approach 10 per cent by the end of the seventies.

Many factors have contributed to this spectacular growth, including: a continuous enlargement of demand for health services, recently augmented by a sizeable expansion of government financing; new methods of financing, including the steady growth of health insurance; scientific and technological advances; and extraordinarily large increases in health care prices.

From the end of World War II to 1966 government outlays hovered steadily around 25 per cent of total expenditures for health. Expenditures of both the public and private sectors were increasing rapidly, but at about the same rate. Within the public sector, state and local governments were spending more than the federal government. The inauguration of major health programs in 1966, particularly Medicare and Medicaid, altered these relationships. Public expenditures reached $22.6 billion in fiscal year 1969 and represented 37.5 per cent of the total. Of this amount about two-thirds was federal money.

Private health insurance was a $1.2 billion annual business in 1950. In fiscal year 1969, it accounted for $13.5 billion, of which $11.7 billion went for health care and the remainder to administration and overhead. Insurance benefits met 22 per cent of all personal health care expenditures and 35 per cent of private and personal care expenditures.

The relative roles of major sources of expenditures have been significantly altered in recent years. For example, in fiscal year 1949–50 private funds accounted for 75 per cent of all health expenditures, of which consumer direct outlays represented 59 per cent, insurance payments (including expenses for prepayment) only 10 per cent, and

TABLE I. *Expenditures for Health and Medical Care, Selected Years 1928–29 through 1968–69 (Dollar Amounts in Millions)*

Type of Expenditure	1928–29	1939–40	1949–50	1959–60	1965–66	1966–67	1967–68	1968–69[1]
Total (dollars)	3,589.1	3,804.6	12,129.5	26,366.7	42,286.2	48,193.3	53,868.6	60,311.9
Private Expenditures	3,112.0	3,023.0	9,064.0	19,971.5	31,464.5	32,315.0	34,158.0	37,701.0
Health & Medical Services	3,010.0	2,992.0	8,812.0	19,326.5	30,136.5	30,932.0	32,653.0	35,981.0
Medical Research	0.0	0.0	37.0	121.0	169.0	175.0	180.0	185.0
Medical-facilities construction	102.0	31.0	215.0	524.0	1,159.0	1,208.0	1,325.0	1,535.0
Public Expenditures	477.1	781.6	3,065.3	6,395.2	10,821.7	15,878.3	19,710.6	22,610.9
Health & Medical Services	372.5	679.5	2,470.2	5,346.3	8,702.2	13,727.4	17,256.3	20,120.6
Medical Research	0.0	2.6	72.9	471.2	1,375.8	1,428.7	1,615.5	1,549.4
Medical-facilities construction	104.7	99.6	522.3	577.7	743.7	722.2	838.9	940.9
Total Expenditures as a per cent of Gross National Product	3.6	4.0	4.6	5.3	5.9	6.2	6.5	6.7
Public Expenditures as a per cent of Total Expenditures	13.3	20.5	25.3	24.3	25.6	32.9	36.6	37.5
Personal Care Expenditures[2]	3,272.2	3,501.7	10,549.4	23,236.2	36,397.7	41,594.0	46,916.9	52,564.3
Private Expenditures	2,990.0	2,979.0	8,447.0	18,306.5	28,511.5	29,143.0	30,756.0	33,835.0
Public Expenditures	282.0	522.7	2,102.4	4,929.7	7,886.2	12,451.0	16,160.9	18,729.3
Per cent from:								
Private Expenditures	91.4	85.1	80.1	78.8	78.3	70.1	65.6	64.4
Direct payments	88.6[3]	82.8[3]	67.7	56.3	51.8	45.8	41.7	40.6
Insurance Benefits	0.0	0.0	8.3	20.2	24.5	22.5	22.2	22.3
Public Expenditures	8.6	14.9	19.9	21.2	21.7	29.9	34.4	35.6

[1] Preliminary estimates.
[2] Includes all expenditures for health services and supplies other than: expenses for prepayment and administration (except in 1928–29 and 1939–40); government public health activities; expenditures of private voluntary agencies for other health services. Includes any insurance benefits and expenses for prepayment (insurance premiums less insurance benefits).
[3] Includes any insurance benefits and expenses for prepayment (insurance premiums less insurance benefits).
Source: Division of Health Insurance Studies, Office of Research and Statistics, Social Security Administration.

the remainder, mainly philanthropy, was 6 per cent. By fiscal 1968–69 the relative position of private funds declined to 62 per cent, of which consumer direct payments were 35 per cent, insurance 22 per cent, and all other 5 per cent.

Types of Expenditure

There has been a substantial shift in the distribution of expenditures among different types of services, reflecting the changing technology of care. Until the end of the thirties, physicians' services accounted for the largest single share. By 1940 hospitals had moved in front and they have increased their share steadily since. Between 1940 and 1968 hospitals moved from 26 per cent to 36 per cent of the health dollar. (Up to this point data have been presented for fiscal years. In the ensuing discussion, the figures are for calendar years.) Primarily as a consequence of extraordinary increases in hospital expenditures, resulting from both the exceptionally high rise in hospital prices and increased use, most of the other categories have declined proportionately. Physicians in private practice moved from 25 per cent to 20 per cent; dentists from 11 per cent to 6 per cent. However, some categories have increased significantly indicating other changing emphases in health care. Nursing home care, which was too small to be reported in 1940, amounted to 4 per cent of the total in 1968. Medical research, for which a virtually negligible sum was spent in 1940, moved up to 3 per cent.

The relation of private and public outlays varies greatly among the different services. Half of the public funds expended for health care in 1968 went for hospital care, but only three-tenths of the private money was spent for this purpose. Nursing home care accounted for less than 2 per cent of private expenditures, but 8 per cent of public outlays. On the other hand, 16 per cent of the private health dollar was spent for out-of-hospital drugs, but only 1 per cent of the public funds.

Elements of Cost

Part of the steady increases in total national expenditures is attributable to the growth of population. This factor is readily eliminated by presenting expenditures on a per capita basis. An average of $29 was spent for every man, woman and child in the population in 1940; $147 in 1960; and $280 in 1968. This indicates an increase of 865 per cent over 29 years, 90 per cent for the last eight years.

Changing prices contributed greatly to this rise. This factor can be eliminated by converting per capita expenditures for each year to constant 1968 dollars by means of the medical care component of the Consumer Price Index. Per capita constant dollars spent more than tripled from 1940 to 1968; increased 70 per cent between 1950 and 1968; and 42 per cent from 1960.

This increase represents in large part a growth in per capita utilization of health services. Part of it may also indicate higher quality of care, although much of this factor may be reflected in the price level which has already been accounted for. Thus utilization appears to show an average annual increase of 3 per cent since 1950 and 4 per cent since 1960, both impressive compounded rates.

The reasons for increased demand despite escalating price levels are multiple. Larger incomes is one factor, but the demand has grown far greater than income alone could explain. Other contributing factors include: changing demographic composition, such as the relative increase of women in the population, especially at older ages; the higher educational levels and resulting greater health consciousness; urbanization of the population; a shift in morbidity patterns from predominance of acute episodic illness to more expensive long-term ailments; increased public support of health care for the poor; and growth of insurance and other third-party payments. Perhaps the single most important element has been the spectacular advance in medical technology, which within this century revolutionized medical care from a service of generally dubious efficacy to one regarded as a life-saving and life-enhancing essential.

Whatever the relative mix of these and other factors, Americans are conspicuously expressing their desire for more and improved health services, pressing against a supply that appears to have fallen far behind in quantity or structural adequacy, or both. Prominent among the frustrations that have accompanied the growing demand is spiraling prices. As we have noted, much of the large increase in per capita expenditures was washed away by price inflation.

Despite substantial growth in individual use of services, price rise has been a greater factor in increasing costs during the post World War II period. Its comparative importance has grown larger in recent years. Professor Victor Fuchs has reported the complex matter in perhaps its simplest form with a computation showing that for the twenty-year period ending 1966, prices increased at an annual rate of 3.7 per cent while use per capita rose 2.7 per cent. In the same period he calculates that per capita income increased 2.3 per cent while per capita expenditures for health services grew 6.4 per cent a year.

The most exhaustive recent analysis examines separately each of the three major categories of expenditure (short-term voluntary hospital care, physicians' services, and dental services), and applies appropriate measures of price increases to each category. Acknowledging the short-comings of available data, the authors (Herbert Klarman, Dorothy P. Rice, Barbara S. Cooper, H. Louis Stetler, in a paper presented to the American Public Health Association, November 11, 1969) show that over the long period, 1929–68, prices contributed one-half the increase in expenditures, population growth about one-sixth, and per capita use (which includes the quality of services) about one-third.

The depression period, 1929–40, was the only time when prices played a less significant role than per capita use; both declined in that period. During the three-year period 1965–68, population accounted for 9 per cent of growth in total expenditures, per capita use for 17 per cent, while increased prices were responsible for 74 per cent.

The picture varies among the three services. During the period 1929–68, the increase in prices accounted for 61 per cent of the growth in short-term hospital expenditures. In recent years, 1965–68, the relative contribution of the price increase has been much greater, 82 per cent. Over the long period price rises accounted for 39 per cent of the increase in expenditures for physicians' services. In recent years they have been responsible for between 50 and 75 per cent of the increased cost. For dental services, price rises accounted for 44 per cent of the increase in total expenditures for the long period and for about 54 per cent in the recent period.

Price Movements

Of course, prices have been going up everywhere. Price rise in the general economy has contributed to the inflation of medical prices. But the differential between general price and health care price increases during the past two decades has been pronounced and persistent. From 1946 to 1969 medical care prices advanced 155 per cent while the index of all prices advanced 88 per cent, an average annual increase of 4.2 per cent versus 2.8 per cent. By far the major influence was hospital daily service charges, which increased 592 per cent, almost seven times as fast as all prices and almost five times as fast as all services in the Consumer Price Index.

For years it was optimistically said that this was in large part a catching-up process, since medical prices had fallen behind other prices during the Great Depression and hospital wages were making up their lag behind other wage scales. After a reasonable period, the argument ran, we could expect a levelling out, and medical price increases would then be generally consistent with other price movements. The prediction has proved invalid. In recent years, as Table II demonstrates, the differential has actually widened significantly. The year 1969 was an exception because general prices experienced an extraordinary inflation of 5.4 per cent. But even then medical care prices rose more sharply, 6.9 per cent.

Cost measurement and price indexes in the health field are far from precision instruments and can be easily faulted conceptually and technically, but the magnitude and consistency of the rises shown by every available measure are so generally uniform and so great that they cannot be explained away by statistical shortcomings, and there can be little doubt about the validity of the general trends indicated.

Health Insurance

Significant steps have been taken to spread the risks and thus reduce the individual burdens of high costs, particularly through the development of private health insurance and government programs. Private health insurance is mainly a post World War II development, given considerable impetus by the threat of President Truman's proposal for compulsory national health insurance. Its growth was spectacular during the fifties. Currently, about four-fifths of the population under age 65 have some form of private health insurance, although with widely varying degrees of protection.

The Medicare program relieved insurance carriers of the almost prohibitive task of adequately insuring the aged, a high-cost low-income population. The apparent inability of the insurance industry to successfully reach remaining portions of the low-income population continues to be an important unresolved issue. Twenty per cent of the civilian population was still wholly unprotected in 1968. That represented more than 36 million persons. A disproportionate number were among the poor and among children.

The proportion of people protected varies directly with income class and, except at higher income levels, with age. Nintety-two per cent of persons in families with incomes of $10,000 or more had some insurance in 1968, but only 36 per cent of those in families with incomes

TABLE II. *Consumer Price Index and Selected Medical Components; Selected Years, 1946–68; Average Annual Indexes and Percentage Changes (1957–59 = 100)*

Type of Expenditure	Price Index						Average Annual Percentage Change			
	1946	1960	1965	1967	1968	1969	1946–60	1960–65	1965–69	1968–69
CPI, all items	68.0	103.1	109.9	116.3	121.2	127.7	3.0	1.3	3.8	5.4
Less medical care	—[1]	102.8	109.1	115.0	119.7	126.1	—[1]	1.2	3.7	5.3
CPI, all services	63.9	105.6	117.8	127.7	134.3	143.7	3.7	2.2	5.1	7.0
Less medical services	—[1]	106.2	116.2	124.7	130.8	139.7	—[1]	1.8	4.7	6.8
Medical care, total	60.7	108.1	122.3	136.7	145.0	155.0	4.2	2.5	6.1	6.9
Medical care services	58.4	109.1	127.1	145.6	156.3	168.9	4.6	3.1	7.4	8.1
Hospital daily service charges	37.0	112.7	153.3	200.1	226.6	256.0	8.3	6.3	13.7	13.0
Physicians' fees	66.4	106.0	121.5	137.6	145.3	155.4	3.4	2.8	6.4	7.1
Dentists' fees	67.0	104.7	117.6	127.5	134.5	143.9	3.2	2.4	5.2	7.0
Drugs and prescriptions[2]	74.6	102.3	98.1	97.9	98.1	99.2	2.3	0.8	0.3	1.1

[1] Not available.
[2] Index base for prescriptions, March 1960; for over-the-counter items, December 1963.
Source: U.S. Bureau of Labor Statistics.

under $3000 and 57 per cent in families with incomes between $3000
and $5000. Only 75 per cent of all children under age 17 were covered
by some insurance. In families with less than $3000 income only 23
per cent of the children had coverage; in families with $3000 to $5000
income it was 49 per cent. It is generally agreed that a great deal more
could be done to correct this situation.

INSURANCE PROTECTION MEAGER

The relatively high numbers of persons with some insurance can
easily produce false comfort. The protection for most people is relatively meager. The rise of third-party payments in recent years has
resulted mainly from government expenditures. Government payments
as a proportion of personal health care expenditues grew from 21
per cent in 1965 to 35 per cent in 1968. Consequently, the portion paid
by private health insurance declined, from 25 per cent to 23 per cent.
Direct consumer payments represented 41 per cent of the total in 1968.

Probably a more informative comparison is the relative role of
insurance in *total consumer* expenditures for personal health care,
omitting all government outlays. Insurance met 32 per cent of consumer expenses in 1965 and 36 per cent in 1968. Out-of-pocket payments were still producing about two-thirds of consumer expenditures.
Insurance payments were heavily skewed among different services.
Insurance benefits met 74 per cent of consumer expenditures for hospital care, 38 per cent of those for physicians' services, and a mere
4 per cent for all other types of care. (Some expenditures for personal
health care probably should not be covered by insurance, such as
expenditures for nonprescribed drugs and the cost of private room
accommodations when not medically necessary. It has been estimated
by Louis S. Reed in the *Social Security Bulletin*, December 1969, that
if such expenditures were deducted from consumer health expenditures,
the proportion of the remainder then met by insurance would be
three or four percentage points higher.)

Insurance has greatly improved access to medical care, especially
for employed workers and their families, since the large majority of
protection is bought through employee-benefit group insurance plans.
By increasing the total volume of money available as well as spreading
payments over a larger population and a sharing of costs by employers,
health insurance has brought the benefits of modern medicine to a
far greater number of people than would otherwise have been possible.
It has also been a financial boon to providers of services. But the
large achievements of health insurance have, with the passage of
time and changing conditions, also developed a host of serious dif-

ficulties. Its future has begun to appear somewhat uncertain. Its own successes contributed to the rising public expectations that it is now having difficulty meeting. The cost crisis it helped stave off in the past appears to be catching up with it.

To meet public expectations and needs, the insurance industry will have to find means to enroll a larger proportion of the population, particularly to reach relatively lower income classes more effectively. It has become clear that Medicaid type of welfare programs now require encompassing too large a segment of the population to permit administrative effectiveness or public acceptance. Medical indigence has proved to be far more widespread than was assumed a few years ago.

BROADER BENEFITS NEEDED

One of the most serious challenges to health insurance is the need for more comprehensive benefits, covering a larger proportion of family medical costs. The problem has two phases. For a long time health insurance has been widely accused of aggravating cost inflation by its imbalance in benefit coverage, which was originally concentrated almost entirely on hospital care and contributed to inappropriate and expensive patterns of utilization. Since people were covered for expenses incurred in a hospital, but not for care outside, a strong tendency developed for use of hospitals even when care of a less expensive kind was equally or more appropriate. Despite recent progress in development of policies designed to render broader protection, the major emphasis still remains on services provided in a hospital, and ambulatory care remains relatively uncovered. While no definitive data are available, it is probable that over 80 per cent of all insurance benefits are paid for hospital-related care. Physicians also point out that restrictive health insurance may have deleterious effects on the quality of care.

The second phase of the problem is in the allegation that not only does the lack of comprehensive coverage cause unbalanced and expensive patterns of utilization, but that it makes unfeasible an adequate level of overall protection. Very large segments of personal health care costs now generally fall in uncovered categories. As indicated earlier, private health insurance meets only four per cent of consumer expenditures for all health services other than those for hospital care and physicians' service. The physicians' services included in most policies do not cover office or home visits.

Although consumers have been rapidly increasing their expenditures for health insurance, the proportion of consumer expense met by insurance has advanced at a very slow pace. In the past decade the increase has averaged slightly more than one percentage point a year and, as we have already noted, the 1968 figure is only a little more than a third of consumer expenditures. At that rate, it would require another 30 years before some two-thirds of consumer expenditures would be covered, a goal that most experts regard as reasonable. The benefits available to Medicare beneficiaries are far more extensive than those currently available to most people with private insurance. The inadequacy of private insurance has thus become more conspicuous and vulnerable.

Several high-level study commissions have recommended legislative action to require a minimum range of benefits in all health insurance sold. Some leaders of the industry have recognized the seriousness of the problem and are now increasingly urging insurers to make policies more comprehensive, to place more emphasis in their coverage on ambulatory care, and to relate their coverage to the encouragement of preventive services.

However, insurance is also a victim of medical price inflation. If carriers are to broaden the range of benefits, they must raise premiums. If to meet rising prices, premiums must be raised ten per cent or more each year just to finance the same package of benefits (the services that most health insurance cover have been experiencing the greatest degree of price inflation), it obviously becomes that much more difficult to tack on still higher premiums for enlarged benefits. In fact, there is evidence that some carriers are being forced to retreat; deductibles and coinsurance, which add to consumers' out-of-pocket expenses, are becoming more common, even though carriers are aware that this opens up another set of complications.

Nonetheless there is considerable evidence to indicate that when consumers are given a choice, they will select broader coverage. This is particularly true when an employer shares the cost.

REDUCE INSURANCE COSTS AND EXPAND ENROLLMENT

There are a number of possible steps the industry could take both to reduce the cost of insurance and enhance the chances of expanding enrollment. Of the 1968 gross total enrollment in health insurance (the gross includes a substantial number of duplicating policies held by the same persons), some 21 per cent held individual policies sold by insurance companies. Premiums paid by individual policy holders represented over one-fourth of the premiums of insurance companies (as distinguished from Blue Cross-Blue Shield and independent plans).

Characteristically such policies are relatively expensive and their protection meager. Under their group business, insurance companies used 93.8 per cent of total earned premium income for benefit payments (about the same as Blue Cross-Blue Shield), but on individual policies, the companies used only 53.6 per cent of premium income for benefits, and that was better than they had done the year before. Over 46 per cent of the premium dollar was never translated into health care, even though the companies sustained a slight net underwriting loss.

Far greater enterprise can be undertaken to convert much of this unfortunate portion of the business into group policies and at the same time enable persons now ineligible for group purchases, and who hold no policies at all, to join groups at the far more attractive rates. For example, it would appear entirely possible to permit the self-employed to enjoy group rates by contriving viable and appropriate groupings by use of associations, geographical, or other bases. Similarly, it would be advantageous if carriers did not experience rate very small groups, wherein one catastrophic illness can make the group rates impractical to sustain. The experience of small groups could be pooled until an account could stand reasonably on its total experience, thus making the small groups less vulnerable.

Employee-benefit plans could be required to include coverage of employees over lay-off periods, say for 90 days, as members of the employed group. This would simply be extending a fringe benefit to conform in part with what is already accepted in principle on basic pay through unemployment compensation.

It is generally believed that a considerable share of all insurance company individual policies are supplementary to other coverages. If the range and adequacy of basic policies were enlarged, as previously suggested, this would reduce the need for purchase of expensive and socially undesirable individual policies. Many other examples could be suggested.

In short, it appears that the possibilities of private health insurance have not yet been sufficiently exploited, and time is now a critical factor. The industry may not find it possible to move effectively in such directions without some limitation being imposed upon the number and character of companies operating in this field—elimination of mail order houses, for example. It may perhaps require that Congress reclaim from the states jurisdiction over insurance regulation. The future of the public-private mix in our pluralistic health economy, indeed whether the financing system remains pluralistic at all, may largely be determined by developments in this area in the near future.

Government Stakes

Governments at all levels spent $21.2 billion for medical care in 1968, about $17.5 billion of it for personal health services, the large bulk of which was provided by the federal government or stimulated by it under grant-in-aid programs. Government's relative share of all health care expenditures rose from 25 per cent to 37 per cent in three years. Much of this growth was the result of Medicare and Medicaid programs. Medicare expenditures were $6 billion in 1968. The vendor medical program of public assistance, primarily Medicaid, paid out $4 billion in 1968 (about half of which came from state and local governments) but only $1.5 billion in 1965.

Cost inflation has been severely felt by government programs. Medicare and Medicaid are exceeding anticipated costs mainly because of greater price rises than seemed reasonable to allow for in earlier estimates. For the hospital insurance part of Medicare, Congress very early had to raise the projected long-term tax rate. The deductible and coinsurance paid by the patient have been increased twice within two years, a total of 30 per cent. Premiums for the supplementary medical insurance part of the program have also been increased twice, by a total of 77 per cent.

On the outlay side, Medicaid benefits have been cut back in a number of states, and Congress introduced restrictive limits on income levels for eligibility the year after the program went into effect. There is widely publicized dissatisfaction with the program for a variety of reasons, but much of it stems from soaring costs. In both programs, the administration has cut back on its payment formulas to providers of care, and the latter have accused the government of welching on its obligations.

The outlook for the future has produced consternation in government circles. Consumer dissatisfactions are increasingly articulated and pressed upon both Congress and the administration. Projections into the future portend budgetary crises from medical costs. If current trends are unabated, by 1975 Medicaid expenditures could consume all of H.E.W.'s anticipated additional appropriations, thus depriving it of new initiatives in its wide range of other responsibilities and depriving it of priority judgments. Moreover, government finds that its great additional expenditures have not only failed to produce equitable utilization of health care resources by the whole population but that there has been small net gain. H.E.W.'s report on the health of the nation's health care system spoke of the "crippling inflation in medical costs causing vast increases in government health expenditures for little return, raising private health insurance premiums and reducing the purchasing power of the health dollar of our citizens."

It has also become clear from government reports that its programs have failed to supply the medical needs of the poor and the black community. Public programs reach only a minority of the 40 million poor and near-poor, as officially defined, and there is considerable question about the extent of the need met even among those who are reached. Medicare is aimed at the aged and therefore does reach a group in which there is heavy concentration of poor and near-poor. Medicaid reached slightly more than 8 million people in 1969, about one-fifth of the poor and near-poor. But of the total Medicaid budget, about 46 per cent goes to the elderly, although they represent only about one-third of the recipients, presumably to cover gaps arising from the fact that Medicare pays for an average of only 45 per cent of health care expenditures of the aged. Other public programs for the poor—such as Office of Economic Opportunity programs and the maternal and child health program—are relatively small. If the 2 million children who received service under Medicaid are added to the 400,000 under maternal and child health programs (disregarding overlaps), we find about 2.5 million children being compared to the 19 or 20 million children among the poor and near poor, about one child out of eight. The administration is sensitive to the social and political implications of these facts but faces the frustrations of high-flying costs.

All of this has resulted in substantial soul-searching in government, as it has in the insurance industry and among some providers of care. There is grave doubt being cast upon the allocation of government resources in this area: doubt, for example, about whether it is equitable or wise that about one-half of all government payments for personal health care is spent for the aged (about one-eighth of government payments are for children under fifteen); and more fundamental reservations about the division of expenditures between purchase of services and building an adequate supply capacity—a difficulty perceived to characterize the entire health care economy as well.

Shortages, tensions, and imbalance pervade the health field. But in 1968 only twenty per cent of federal expenditures for health were directed at investment in categories designed to improve or augment supply, and more than half of that went for support of biomedical research. In the budget for fiscal year 1970 investment in such categories dropped to sixteen per cent of total federal outlays. Government authorities readily admit that since 1966 government has been a major contributor to the imbalance between demand and supply.

But it has become clear that the sources of the multitude of apparent difficulties in health care are more complex and deeper than the multiplication of demand. In any case, the government could not retreat from its support of consumption; on the contrary, all indications are that it may be obliged to enlarge it. Nor is there any probability that privately financed demand will be abated. Moreover, the rapid increase of costs has considerably curtailed leeway for allocation of more funds to augment supply under tight budgetary conditions, especially with rising resistance against pouring more money into a supply system that is widely believed to be using resources wastefully and at relatively low levels of productivity. There is growing sentiment that if new investment in supply is to be effective, it must be related to a redesigned delivery structure.

Sources of Cost Rise

As already indicated, prices appear to have been the most important element in cost rise in recent years, at least in relation to the two major services, hospital care and physicians' services. Explanations for the extraordinary price inflation are controversial. Different sectors of providers operate differently and are subject to different influences. The price behavior of the several sectors varies. Space considerations require that we confine our discussion here to hospitals, the largest sector and the one in which price rise has been most pronounced.

HOSPITAL COST RISE JUSTIFICATIONS

Prominent among the more frequent justifications advanced for acceleration hospital costs are:

1. Medical and hospital technology have been advancing at a phenomenal pace with commensurate demands on facilities, equipment, personnel, and services. Those admitted use more services per capita, such as diagnostic and therapeutic X-ray procedures, drugs, and laboratory services. There has been a growth in the range of services made available. For example, between 1963 and 1968 the proportion of community hospitals with intensive care services (including coronary care services) jumped from 18 per cent to 42 per cent. The equipment for all such services grows more elaborate and costly, and its rate of obsolescence more rapid.

2. The rise in labor costs is conspicuous. A by-product of advancing technology has been additional and more specialized personnel. Also, hospitals have been gradually catching up with long overdue improvements in wages and working conditions. Reduction in hours of work has caught up with other industries. A lag still exists in wages and the next few

years will probably witness through law and bargaining an equalization between hospital and similar types of employment. Many hospital officials assert that when this occurs, hospital prices will stabilize in relation to other prices.

3. Hospitals have assumed increased functions in addition to direct patient care. Important among these is education. Despite the decline in hospital-based schools of nursing, they still account for about four-fifths of registered nurse graduates, and the cost of these programs to the hospitals is rising. With federal subsidies for nurse education and the trend toward academic settings for such education, this burden should eventually decline but it will be slow. Also, many hospitals have been adding full-time directors of medical education, an additional, although modest, factor in costs. (Stipends of interns and residents are considered professional service costs rather than education.)

4. Hospital financing is increasingly coming through commercial borrowing, rather rare in the past. Interest charges, still a small part of total operating expenses, are nonetheless adding a new factor to hospital costs.

5. The common measure of hospital prices, the average per diem expenses, is misleading. The factors in the numerator—total operating costs—have less and less relationship to the denominator—inpatient days. Hospitals increasingly engage in a variety of other services and activities; particularly there has been a rapid increase in outpatient services. The American Hospital Association has, therefore, recently developed a different denominator. It takes into account outpatient services by converting them into outpatient day equivalents and deriving an "adjusted patient day" figure. This, of course, reduces the average per diem figure. However, the previously cited study by Klarman and his associates indicates that when this adjustment is carried back in time, the result has no significant effect upon hospital price trends. (It should be noted that Consumer Price Index figures used in this chapter are not based on per diem costs, but upon daily service charges for room, board, and nursing services.)

6. Another factor, perhaps overlapping point 1 above, is the changing mix of patients. Patients with relatively serious illness, requiring the more complex and expensive procedures, represent an increasing proportion of the hospital population.

UNANSWERED HOSPITAL COST RISE QUESTIONS

Critics of hospital costs do not find such explanations satisfying. As statements of fact, they are true, as far as they go. But they do not enlighten one on the extent of the price rise which each, or their aggregate, may explain. Nor do they indicate to what extent the factual developments are justifiable or necessary.

It cannot be questioned that there has been a great expansion of facilities, equipment, personnel, and services. But how much represents unnecesary duplication of facilities and equipment among several hospitals within the same community, because each hospital behaves as an autonomous unit rather than as part of a coordinated health care system? How much of the new equipment are prestige or convenience items?

How much of the mounting increase in ancillary services is simply a result of the spread of third-party payment which has reduced the physician's inhibitions to additional laboratory procedures or an additional day's stay in hospital, and the individual consumer's resistance to higher costs, on which a normal market situation would place considerable reliance?

Has there been any attempt to measure the relative value to health care represented by new equipment and added services, or are "improved models" bought without such criteria because hospitals now have a virtual guarantee of repayment of all their costs from third-party payors? Has there been progress toward developing measures of cost-benefit relationships?

Payrolls have indeed increased and these are, of course, the major factor in hospital operating costs. But it is not true that payroll costs have advanced more rapidly than other costs in recent years. From 1960 to 1968, despite a substantial rise in personnel in relation to patient load, total expenses per patient day advanced more rapidly than payroll per patient day, 90 per cent against 82 per cent. Payrolls accounted for 62 per cent of total expenses in 1960 and 60 per cent in 1968.

Moreover, wage increases cannot be charged with the whole responsibility for payroll increases. The American Hospital Association attributes half of increased total expenditures for wages and salaries between 1963 and 1968 to additional employment. For many years hospitals have been steadily adding more and more personnel per patient. In the last five-year period alone, 1963–1968, the number of employees per 1000 adjusted patient days increased 13 per cent.

The hospitals are accused of an insatiable capacity for absorbing more manpower, the only restraint being their availability. They had an alleged manpower crisis in 1950 when hospitals were employing 178 persons per 100 inpatients; now there are 272 employees per 100 inpatients—a striking increase of 53 per cent which cannot be fully explained by the growth of outpatient services—and a manpower crisis is even more loudly proclaimed. There are wide variations in the personnel-patient ratios among states, but there are no indications of any correlation with quantity of care received or health results.

LAG IN PRODUCTIVITY

A major issue thus lies in the hospital's apparent failure or inability to employ new technology for productivity increases, which has characterized the rest of the American economy. Introduction of new equipment and procedures has been accompanied by more rather than less personnel. In fact, hospitals justify additional personnel by such developments.

Such data do not prove anything definitively, because quality—one element in productivity—has undoubtedly risen. But how much or in what degree it is comparable to the rise in personnel or other resources is not known. Nevertheless there appears some basis for a presumption that net productivity is falling or, at best, is static. One may concede that a labor-intensive personal service industry will have more difficulty improving productivity than will manufacturing firms. While precise parallels are never available, some other service industries—for example, financial institutions—have demonstrated that very significant gains can be made. Is it really impossible in hospitals? Or is there a lack in incentives, in skills, or in organizational structure that is inhibiting? Perhaps it is the eleemosynary tradition, or perhaps the persistent myths built around the special character of the service, that fosters the widely held notion that efficiency and concern for productivity are enemies of quality, a problem that prevails in education as well. The contrary is likely to be true. Effective quality control and cost control generally go hand in hand.

In a field notably lacking in satisfactory measures of unit costs, definitions of output, productivity, or effectiveness, neither side in the debate can prove its position conclusively. But the circumstantial evidence is great that the cost aberrations are an important symptom of basic organizational shortcomings. This is underpinned by increasing professional conviction that the delivery structure is obsolete and ineffective from a quality viewpoint as well. Thus, interestingly, those approaching the problem from the perspective of cost efficiency and those attacking it from a quality effectiveness view appear to have arrived at very similar sets of reform proposals. The two objectives are consonant.

A large number of distinguished commissions, study groups, and task forces have looked into virtually all aspects of health care and its costs and made numerous recommendations. They are far too many even to be enumerated here, let alone described. It may, however, be useful to call brief attention to a few broad trends that appear to be developing, although most are still vaguely defined and all quite fragmentary. It is not possible to say how much general agreement any of these have won, but each has received considerable attention in responsible circles, and they appear to point the general direction of the emerging future. Implicitly or explicitly, they also indicate widely held beliefs regarding causes of high costs.

The reform trends, although multiple, can, like the criticisms, be said to fall into two broad classes: improvements in the delivery system, its organization and management; and changes in financing arrangements. The two overlap at many points. It is now better understood than it was only a decade ago that the character of financing influences the delivery system and vice versa.

Systemization

At its best our medical care product can be superb, but it is often very poor. It has been colorfully described by Dr. Peter Rogatz as a technically excellent product thrown into a Rube Goldberg delivery contraption which distorts and defeats it, and makes it more expensive than it need be, because "we do not have a health care *system*—we have a *happening*, with everyone 'doing his own thing.' " The eminent Barr Committee (H.E.W. Secretary's Advisory Committee on Hospital Effectiveness, 1968) reported that "The key fact about the health service as it exists today is this disorganization. . . . lack of planning and control in the health services has resulted in fragmentation and disjunction that promote extravagance and permit tragedy."

It has often been pointed out that in the typical American community the various health service resources have little organizational relationship to one another. Individual hospitals are autonomous in their structure and decision-making. Services and equipment may be duplicated unnecessarily, and costly surpluses may abound in several institutions. Other necessary services may be available in none. Excess of facilities for highly sophisticated types of procedures can be dangerous as well as costly. Some hospitals, partly because of the competitive search for prestige, have built and staffed such units (cardiovascular surgery is a not uncommon example) for which there turns out to be an insufficient case load; the staff is thus unable to maintain the skills necessary for optimum performance. Other health institutions in the community—clinics and skilled nursing homes—may or may not have any organizational relationship with a hospital or with one another. A physician may have some affiliation with one or several hospitals (in some cases, none) and for some parts of his practice it may prove to be the wrong hospital. Organization has not been adapted to mesh the efforts of increased specialisms.

For the patient this fragmentation often means confusion, uncertainty, disjunction, and lack of comprehensiveness in care. Access to appropriate level and site of care is limited by the dispersion of specialized professional personnel and facilities. Quality is restricted by gaps in available services, lack of a point of responsibility for the patient as a whole, and discontinuity of care. Productivity is curtailed by the inherent waste of such dispersion and lack of integration, and cost is increased.

The objective is to bring together the bits and pieces into a system which relates them to one another organizationally, and thus illuminates the gaps as well as the surpluses. At whatever point a patient enters the system—the physician's office, outpatient department of a hospital, or a clinic—the organized system should have responsibility for equal access to the spectrum of services—preventive, diagnostic, therapeutic, and rehabilitative—coordinated to maintain a primary doctor-patient relationship, avoid unnecessary duplication of tests and other services, assure that the appropriate level of institutional care is assigned, and provide centralized complete medical records for each patient.

To achieve this goal, a community would have to define the different functions of different institutions from primary care to the specialized sophisticated procedures of a medical center. Among other things, this means development of community health centers (or primary health centers, to remove any poverty connotations) and increased ambulatory services by hospitals. It would require that every physician have a professional relationship with a community hospital or medical center.

It would enable more efficient use of manpower by wider use of paraprofessional personnel. Many of the tasks traditionally carried out by physicians, for example, can be performed as well by others with far less training and at less expense. A coordinated system could adopt performance standards for many levels of personnel, instead of sole dependence upon diplomas, and thus effectuate both vertical and horizontal mobility of personnel where none now exists. More effective employment of existing personnel might reduce the magnitude of alleged manpower shortages.

Planning

System requires planning, and planning to be effective requires controls. The Barr Committee graphically portrayed the kind of situations that have produced a general acknowledgment of the necessity for planning:

Two new hospitals, both half empty, within a few blocks of each other in one city neighborhood; half a dozen hospitals in another city equipped and staffed for open heart surgery, when the number of cases would barely keep one of the centers busy; empty beds the rule rather than the exception in obstetrical and pediatric services across the nation; aged, chronically ill patients lying idle in $60-a-day hospital beds because no nursing home beds are provided; overloaded emergency rooms, and under-used facilities and services that have been created for reasons of prestige rather than need.

The Hill-Burton Act of 1946 was the nation's first attempt at a very limited form of planning, related to hospital construction using federal financial assistance. Starting in 1960, the U.S. Public Health Service began to render financial support to local and state planning groups, generally voluntary nongovernmental bodies. They interpreted their task to pass on proposals for new construction or expansion of health institutions in terms of the needs of the area of jurisdiction. The bodies generally lacked any formal authority, and most were of very limited effectiveness.

Recently, the concept of planning has broadened to encompass an organized attempt to introduce rationality in relationships among the autonomous entities in health care, to move toward a coordinated system of facilities and personnel hopefully enabled to offer comprehensive services to a given area. From a negatively oriented function of saying no to unnecessary facilities, its mission is now viewed as an affirmative sponsoring of the development of an effective mix of services in an efficient framework. It would provide a mechanism for allocation of area resources to maximize output and accessibility. As one writer put it, it would create a technostructure for what is now essentially a cottage industry.

Presumably, the Partnership for Health legislation enacted by Congress in 1965 (P.L. 89-749) was intended to establish machinery in each state for such goals. Health planning councils have been established all over the nation. For the most part, they have been ineffectual. Their functions have not been clearly defined either by Washington or the states and most of the councils are faltering on the unresolved question of what it is they are expected to do. The councils are local or state voluntary groups without an adequate administrative framework. They lack legal enforcement powers.

Mandatory Planning

Clearly, a new structure for planning is required. It would be tragic if, at a time when virtually all the major affected interests appear ready to turn to planning to cope with major health care issues, the idea should become discredited only because the presently ill-conceived legislation is not functioning. It is now generally agreed that in the absence of a market regulator and discipline, a source of external regulation and control must be substituted. Several states have, in varying degrees, established modest regulatory mechanisms, including New York, California, and Rhode Island. The Secretary of Health, Education and Welfare has asked Congress for legislation which would make Medicare reimbursement contingent upon prior approval of the facility in question by the appropriate geographic planning body, if and when such a body becomes effective in a particular locale. The same bill would require that every individual institution have an institutional plan respecting its own activities, in recognition of the fact that effective community planning must start at the level of the individual institution. The American Hospital Association has officially accepted the principle of mandatory planning (although conditioned upon a quid pro quo of third-party payors accepting responsibility for capital financing in its reimbursement formulas). Blue Cross plans have said they "will not pay full reimbursement or continue our contract" with hospitals that do not comply with health planning agencies. Commercial carriers have taken a sympathetic stance. A report ("Health Care Delivery in the 1970's," Committee on Medical Economics, Health Insurance Association of America, October 1969) says:

> The cost of building, equipping, and maintaining a modern hospital has become so great, that it is no longer economical to use such an institution for convalescent care or the treatment of chronic illnesses, to say nothing of custodial care. . . .

> While there is no agreement on the "proper" number of general hospital beds per thousand population, there is agreement that, whatever the number, both hospital administrators and physicians will see that the beds are kept filled. This suggests that a moratorium should be declared on building new hospital beds until the need for more beds, or such an expensive type, can be fully justified. In particular, the "two beds per thousand population" rule of thumb used by many prepaid group practice plans should be checked for validity, since it is so significantly lower than the national average of about four per thousand.

It appears that the parties at interest are ready for effective action, but machinery is sadly lacking. It also seems clear that if the machinery is to be effective, the agencies will have to be given enforcement powers. Their range of functions will require changes in existing restrictive legislation in the states. For example, as the Health Insurance Association of America has noted, there is

. . . virtually unanimous agreement that the present rigid guild system applicable to nurses aids, nurses, and other paramedical personnel should be eliminated, so that individuals with the talent and perseverance to do so may advance up the ladder of a health care career through on-the-job training or taking of additional courses. . . . Licensing laws and regulations will also have to be changed in most instances.

Such change is essential for better deployment of available personnel resources to help meet the current shortages.

Other licensure laws for health providers and facilities are obsolete and run counter to present-day health requirements. Obviously hospital licensing must be compatible with the standards of the authorized planning agency; franchising may have to be substituted for licensing. Laws in many states effectively prohibit the development of prepaid group practice plans. These must be repealed.

An effective planning instrumentality also offers the best opportunity for meeting the growing demand for consumer participation in decision-making and consumer education in health care matters when properly designed.

PROPRIETARY HEALTH ORGANIZATIONS

The recent energetic invasion of the hospital field, and other health institutions, by national chains of proprietary organizations has generated a new sense of urgency among community hospitals, in particular, regarding the necessity of the planning process and better controls through more meaningful licensure. The community hospitals fear that these new organizations, because of their methods of doing business, represent a threat to the structure and financing of health services in the community. It is alleged that the chains siphon off only the cream of the hospital business, accepting only relatively simple cases and leaving the complex and expensive patients for the community hospitals. It is also claimed that they leave the entire burden of charity cases, Medicaid patients, and other non-full-payment cases to community hospitals. Since doctors often are required to own stock in these proprietary institutions, they develop a stake in directing profitable cases to those hospitals. All of this will, it is feared, unduly raise prices in community hospitals and make their financing considerably more difficult.

On the other hand, some observers feel the introduction of these high-powered organizations into the hospital field could prove a healthy influence. It is said that a display of the possibilities of business efficiency and organization is sorely needed in a field too long immune from such drives and too long shielded by the claim that only non-profit institutions could insure quality.

Effective community planning and controls ought to be able to reconcile the problem. Proprietary institutions, as well as community hospitals, can be obliged to accept their appropriate share of community-wide health responsibilities in all forms if meaningful licensing tied to effective state and local planning control mechanisms exist, while yet allowing for the innovative advantages derived from the existence of more than one type of hospital.

Prepaid Group Practice Plans

The relative effectiveness of community prepaid group practice plans at comparativly low cost has revived interest in such arrangements. Some of these plans are operating realities encompassing a number of the objectives of the reformers. The better plans offer one-door comprehensive services at a preset annual fee. They enjoy the economies of scale with adequate nonprofessional staffing for bookkeeping and paper work to permit professionals to devote maximum time to their skills. Preventive care is encouraged as it appears advantageous to the plan as well as the patient. Incentives for savings to the plan and better health for the patient are built into the plan as the two are made mutually dependent. Health professionals are encouraged to try new methods and procedures as they share in the savings that improved organization can achieve.

The National Advisory Commission on Health Manpower (1967) made a careful case study of the west coast's Kaiser Foundation Medical Care Program, and described the detailed results in glowing terms for both quality and efficiency:

> The. . . . Program provides comprehensive services to more than a million and a half members drawn primarily from the working population. These services are provided at significant saving by comparison with the cost for equivalent services purchased in the surrounding communities and the country at large. The quality of care provided by Kaiser is equivalent, if not superior, to that available in most communities. . . . Patient satisfaction is indicated by the overall flow of patients into Kaiser from competing health plans under the dual choice available to all Kaiser subscribers.

One of the main sources of economy has been the ability of Kaiser to discourage excessive hospital use. After adjustments were made for age differences, Kaiser subscribers in California were found to have hospitalization rates more than 30 per cent below the state average.

Between 1960 and 1965, hospital patient days of Kaiser subscribers declined by 12 per cent, while those of the United States as a whole increased by 9 per cent. Primarily on this account, the Kaiser plan was able to hold the rise in its expenditures for hospital care during this period to 15 per cent compared to a 50 per cent increase for the United States.

The lower hospital use rates of Kaiser members did not result in higher outpatient medical costs. In fact, the cost of physician services to Kaiser members was appreciably lower than the state average. The staff study concluded that "the average Kaiser member obtains high quality medical care for 20–30 per cent less than the cost of comparable care obtained outside the Plan. . . . the majority of savings achieved by Kaiser results primarily from effective control over the nature of medical care that is provided and over the place where care is given."

The report also found that the experience of the Federal Employees Health Benefits Program, the largest in the nation, using a variety of private health insurance plans, confirms that prepaid comprehensive care plans generally experience hospital use rates lower than any other type of insurance. It explains:

> Almost none of the factors that encourage excessive hospitalization exist in the plans providing comprehensive care. The patients' medical expenses are covered whether incurred inside or outside the hospital; extensive outpatient facilities are available to the physician; the physician is paid on a salary or per capita basis, so that unnecessary hospitalization does not add to his income.

It is therefore not surprising that government is seeking means to encourage the development and use of such plans. Minor legislation has been passed to promote construction of group practice facilities by government guarantees of mortgages. Health insurance carriers appear to be moving toward a similar conclusion. Some leading figures in the industry have stated that to improve productivity, insurers should provide financial assistance for prepaid group practice medical plans.

Managerial Revolution

The heritage of a "charity institution," the anomalous organizational structure, and the relatively small size of the average organization, together with other special features, have resulted in a neglect of efficient management as a recognized responsibility in American hospitals. Attitudes have changed in recent years and a corps of trained professional administrators is appearing. But resistant old traditions and built-in diffusion and ambiguity of authority remain formidable obstacles even to highly skilled administrators. *Fortune* magazine headlined a recent article, "Before We Start a New Building Binge, We Had Better Recognize That Hospitals Need Management Even More Than Money."

The difficulties are both external—the relationship of hospitals and other medical institutions to one another—and internal. The most obvious factor in the external category is the separateness of each institution. About half of all short-term hospitals have fewer than 100 beds, considerably too small to afford or warrant the employment of adequate managerial talent. The lack of skilled personnel managers, for example, is perhaps among the explanations of the notoriously poor labor relations of hospitals. Except among proprietary institutions, mergers are almost unknown. In the not-for-profit sector, the incentives are lacking.

There is no good reason, except in tradition and vested interest, that a group of hospitals should not be under a single management. For communities with only one hospital it would be quite practical for joint management to cover several contiguous communities. The resulting efficiencies and economies of scale could be considerable. Administrators are aware of the advantages, and in some areas arrangements have been made for joint purchasing, joint laundry operations, and the like, which have proved beneficial. But this is not a substitute for unified management. As a by-product, if all hospitals in a community were under single management, present planning difficulties would be minimized. The management plan of such an operation would itself be a very substantial part of the community plan.

Internally there have been great improvements with the gradual professionalization of hospital administration. But the authority of the administrator is severly limited and often ambiguous. The physicians, who typically are not employed by the hospital but are privileged to use its facilities for their patients, generally determine or dominate important hospital policies. Yet the doctors are in an essentially irresponsible position in relation to the efficiency and financing of the hospital. The administrator does not have adequate authority to cope with the prestige or convenience empire-building of the physicians—and sometimes of the trustees as well—who have no personal financial stake in the results. Excessive equipment and costly low occupancy rates (over twenty per cent of the average hospital beds are normally empty) are the consequence. Administrators are frequently appalled by a system which uses expensive beds as freely as we do. One has compared it to "using a Mack truck to deliver a suitcase when a taxicab could do the job as well and a lot cheaper."

The crucial role of managerial effectiveness is now generally recognized and a source of increased concern. Proposals have been made that a minimum standard of managerial adequacy be included among the conditions of participation in Medicare. Others have gone further and recommended that management competence be a condition of licensure.

There is an active search for a formula to provide integrated management. Some medical groups have urged that representatives of the medical staff be appointed to boards of trustees. Leaving aside the potential conflict of interest that can arise from such a design, it would do little to consolidate managerial responsibility in the hospital. The Barr Committee moved closer to the mark in recommending that:

> Appropriate members of the medical staff shall be directly involved with administration in developing the budget and operating plan, and in the achievement of financial and service objectives as budgeted and planned; and

> The institution's financial budget and operating plan shall be reviewed by the board of trustees . . . which shall delegate to the administrator the authority required to enable him to manage the operations of the institution in accordance with the approved financial budget and operating plan.

Payments to Providers

HOSPITAL PAYMENTS

Third-party payments now represent about 90 per cent of hospital revenue for patient care. Government and Blue Cross plans, which are the source of a large majority of this income, generally reimburse on the basis of actual costs. The particular formulas are, of course, always in controversy but both sides have accepted the principle of payments for costs. However, the principle has now fallen into general disrepute as inherently inflationary and as a failure of the payors to meet their fiscal responsibility. The heavy infusion of Medicare and Medicaid money dramatized a problem which had been in operation on a smaller scale for a long time.

The method is accused of generating disincentives for efficiency or economy and in some quarters has been blamed for part of the recent acceleration in price rise. If a hospital has a virtual guarantee of repayment of its costs, where is the motivation to drive for more economical procedures, to resist staff demands for more expensive equipment, or to abstain from adding personnel? Almost everybody now expresses discontent; the philosophy of open-ended retroactive cost reimbursement is no longer defended. But what should be substituted? Here the agreement breaks down; in fact, there are very few positive ideas in circulation on this knotty problem.

In 1967 the Congress authorized Medicare experimentation with different methods of payment to institutions. A small number have recently been started and results will not be available for some time. However, there is only small optimism about their prospects. Most are built around some version of "incentive payments"; an institution that experiences cost saving as measured against a preset target cost, or against some general average of comparable hospitals, is permitted to share in the savings by being paid something more than actual costs. There is some question about the effectiveness of this type of incentive in relation to non-profit voluntary institutions which cannot distribute dividends from such "profits." They can be used for additional perquisites for staff or for capital investment, but this raises questions about long-term effects because such expenditures drive up costs in future years.

"Ceiling rates" are employed in some areas for Blue Cross payments (in New Jersey, for example, where they are set by the State Commissioner of Banking and Insurance), but the arbitrariness of such lines can be destructive and can unwittingly penalize the wrong institutions. Among the more prominent proposals are various versions of prior budget review and advance negotiated rates. While it is generally agreed that rates negotiated between the parties are likely to end up at the level of actual costs, it is felt that it would have the advantages of obliging the institution to defend its budget plans in advance, and permit the payor to assert a disallowance of certain costs, for reimbursement purposes, before the expenditure is made. The payor would also be able to bargain on "reasonableness" of costs in relation to the costs of similarly situated institutions. Aside from the tremendous administrative burden of bargaining annually with thousands of individual hospitals, a frequent objection is that such prior control is likely to have a curbing influence upon innovation, as institutions might be pressed into a preconceived and conventional mold.

Other issues are contained in the question as to what types of expenditures should be reimbursed as a cost of patient care. For example, should the costs of education in hospitals be charged to patient care, as they now generally are, or are these general community obligations to be paid for from public funds or philanthropy? Should reimbursements include an allowance for new capital funds for the institution? While such capital payments do not represent the cost incurred for current patients, they are essential if future patients are to be cared for, say the advocates. The opposition points out that such allowances would not distinguish between institutions that need expansion and those that ought not to expand or perhaps even to renew—unless the funds were channeled into a community planning pool for all health care needs. Moreover, they believe there are better ways of meeting capital needs. If third-party payors were to become responsible for generating new capital, would they also have to take some authority over how such funds were used?

PHYSICIAN PAYMENTS

Methods of paying for physicians' services are under similar challenge, but for different reasons. The general rule for both government and insurance carriers—who together are paying about 52 per cent of physicians' fees—is to pay the "going charge," generally referred to as customary (the physician's usual fee) and prevailing (the common rate in the community). In a seller's market of scarce supply, this too is widely proclaimed to be an invitation to inflation. In the two decades preceding Medicare and Medicaid, physicians' fees rose at an average annual rate of slightly more than 3 per cent. But in each of the three years following, the rate of increase was double or more than the previous rate. Physicians' net incomes have, of course, risen more rapidly since the rate of utilization of their services has also gone up.

The obvious answer is to increase the supply of doctors. Efforts in this direction have been made and the annual number of graduates from medical schools has increased substantially, but even that has only barely succeeded in keeping the ratio of doctors to growing population about constant in recent years. The prospect of even approximately meeting the shortage of doctors through more graduates in the foreseeable future—the government figure for the current shortage is 50,000—is extremely dim, although much can be done to utilize the existing supply more effectively.

Some have suggested attempts to curtail demand. This, in fact, is part of the rationalization for deductibles and coinsurance. In practice, they don't appear to be much of a restraint. If they were, they would then meet the objection that they are a barrier to necessary care and prejudicial against low-income people. Rising prices have clearly not held back demand. On the contrary, the future appears to hold the prospect of larger demand. There is still great unmet need. A more adequate supply of doctors would, for example, almost certainly promote a justifiable increase in utilization among the poor.

There is no scientific answer to the question of whether physicians' fees have risen faster than they "should have," because a large element of individual value judgment must go into any such verdict. The objective evidence merely tells us that the fees have been rising faster than most other prices, and faster than in the past, and that they are uncontrolled. The so-called rise in doctor productivity is not an answer. We have no real measure of productivity; the source of the statement is only that doctors are seeing more patients than before. Since doctors typically already work very long hours and the average work week has apparently reached a high plateau, this means that the average time of a patient visit has been shortened. Are two visits of five minutes each more productive than one of ten minutes? Moreover, it would be argued, the increase in visits should have had the reverse effect since most doctors could have improved their incomes nicely without unusual increases in fees.

In any case, it does seem clear that the normal economic controls of the competitive market place are not operating in medical care. An active examination is under way for substitute controls, resting on the view that government and carriers cannot indefinitely guarantee to pay fees which are essentially unilaterally established by the profession itself. Many variations of fee regulation—bargained, negotiated, or administered—are being widely considered. The hope is to find a balance: to minimize limitations upon physicians while establishing adequate public protection. In addition, there is some discussion of the less promising possibility of finding more effective, yet equitable, consumer financial incentives for restraining utilization.

Universal Health Insurance

We have earlier discussed some of the complaints against the inadequacies of present health insurance protection—its skewing of utilization towards the most expensive form of care, its narrow range of benefits, and its insufficient population coverage. Despite the industry's growing sensitivity to the problem and enlightened pronouncements by some of its leaders, the feeling is spreading that under the economics of the situation it will not be possible for private health insurance alone to meet the problem adequately. Consequently, there has been a marked revival of interest in "national health insurance," with a proliferation of well publicized proposals. The dramatic rise in costs has been a major stimulus.

The term "national health insurance" is being used to label a wide variety of quite different programs whose only common factor is their apparent intent that health insurance be made effectively available to the entire population. Beyond this plans differ in virtually all essentials.

So do the apparent motivations of various sponsoring groups. Some believe that large-scale government financial support is the only practical way of meeting the rising costs for an increasing segment of the population. Others see a national program as the only way to control costs. Some view a unified national program as the means to gain the leverage needed to reorganize the delivery system to achieve optimum quality and effectiveness. Still others see universal coverage as a means to stave off the pressure for changing the system and averting government controls, despite the necessary government subsidy. These and other purposes are, of course, not all mutually exclusive and several may be harbored by the same groups.

TYPES OF UNIVERSAL INSURANCE PROPOSALS

One group of proposals can be generally described as variations on an extension of Medicare to the entire population. Typically, employers and employees would share two-thirds of the cost under a social security type of payroll tax. One-third would be provided from federal general revenues. The proposals generally offer a broader range of benefits than Medicare. The agency administering the program would be responsible for seeing that quality and cost controls and innovation for improving the delivery system were applied. Prominently identified with this type of plan is the Committee for National Health Insurance.

A second category of plans, which is primarily identified with Governor Nelson Rockefeller, would establish, either on a state or federal level, preferably the latter, a requirement that all employers purchase a certain minimum quantity of health insurance for all employees with the employer paying at least 50 per cent of the cost. For low-wage workers and short-term unemployed, there would be a government subsidy to help meet the premiums. For the long-term unemployed and unemployable there would be buy-in arrangements with government funds.

A third group of proposals would offer income tax credits to offset the cost of purchasing health insurance (up to a maximum figure) on a sliding scale of 100 per cent to 25 per cent related to income class. Those whose incomes are too low to pay an income tax would have their premiums paid by government. Purchases would be optional.

Congressman Fulton introduced such a bill, which was endorsed by the American Medical Association (which also has a somewhat different proposal of its own). The legislation would deal only with the cost of insurance and provides no standards for what the insurance would actually buy.

The scope of support for one or another of these and less prominent proposals suggests that the nation is beginning to move towards a consensus that some form of universal insurance is necessary. Yet one can hardly assume that, therefore, legislative action is imminent. Disagreement is very great indeed on the appropriate timing of such action and on the type of program needed.

ANALYSIS OF PROPOSALS

The tax credit type of plan has for many the attraction of minimal government involvement, except for the huge subsidy. It also finds some appeal in that most of the funds, deriving from general revenues, would reflect a more progressive source of taxes than relatively regressive payroll taxes. However, the lack of involvement of any responsible administering body is also its glaring deficiency. Apparently the plan assumes that all is well with the present situation except that more money must be made available for people to pay bills. Nothing is proposed to alter anything in the present structure and no standards are established. It simply provides a government guarantee for payment of premiums. This would seem also to guarantee a substantial stimulus to even greater inflation of prices and costs than we have known.

Since insurance would remain optional, the plan also has the hazard of non-universality and adverse selection of risks. Young, healthy, and optimistic people might not buy insurance even at the bargain rates. Others might not do so out of sheer ignorance.

The second category of plans has little attraction on a state basis, except perhaps in the spirit of using some states as experimental laboratories to test what might prove effective for the nation. A health care program run by individual states is likely to have most of the pitfalls that have discredited Medicaid—wide and inequitable variations in benefits among states, inadequate financial resources in many states, low levels of administrative capacity in some states, resistance to establishing adequate standards for fear of heavier tax burdens than neighboring or other states competing for industry, etc.

It has more attraction as a national plan. It might involve least departure from present patterns of insurance. The bulk of private health insurance is now in employee-benefit plans. However, it suffers from some of the same shortcomings as the tax-credit plans. Although it does provide for a minimum package of benefits (relatively small in the current New York bill), no additional standards and controls for quality are provided.

The first group of plans, the Reuther type, generally offers the most comprehensive range of benefits. It is the only one with assured coverage of the entire population, without distinction, in a uniform program. Although it is vague on specifics, it recognizes the need for improving our methods of providing care, for better quality controls, and for infusing efficiency into the system. It establishes a locus of administrative responsibility. The chief criticism directed at this type of plan is based on a fear of monopolistic control by the federal government. Many people feel there are advantages in the pluralism represented by a variety of competing carriers that ought to be retained. Despite the plan's attempt to provide for decentralized decision-making the anticipation is that essential policies will all emerge from one source and this could prove stultifying. (For a recent proposal that attempts to merge the assets of this type of plan with the advantages of pluralism, modeled after the successful Federal Employees Health Benefits Program, see Anne R. Somers, *National Health Insurance: Major Proposals and Issues,* Paper presented to United Hospital Fund, New York City, January 29, 1970.)

As is usually true in such campaigns, all of the advocates claim more for their plans than is actually provided. For example, all are represented as being able to do away with the need for Medicaid and welfare-type medical assistance programs. As none of the proposals would pay 100 per cent of health care costs, such a result is unlikely. The degree of reduction in medical assistance programs would, of course, vary with the extent of benefit coverage. Some of the plans might leave us with the anomaly of a substantial assistance program operating in the presence of so-called national health insurance.

TIMING OF NATIONAL INSURANCE PLAN

The timing issue has divided even those otherwise in agreement on program. The fear, expressed by spokesmen of the Nixon administration among many others, is that unless great corrections are made in the supply situation, the vast infusion of demand generated by universal coverage could cause a breakdown in the entire system. Advocates of early action, particularly those who support a Reuther-type proposal, do not deny the dangers in the stringency of supply. They generally argue that the dangers are great even now and only with the authority and incentive of a national plan will it be possible to tackle the supply problem meaningfully and adequately, and this they intend to do.

The other side expresses the opposite fear, that a pumping of massive amounts of new money into the system by government would underpin the present arrangements and induce a recurrence of public apathy. By removing the current pressures we may be removing the best leverage we have for necessary change. This group also points to the lack of specificity in the Reuther program regarding the means that would be employed to regulate the system. It doubts the practicality of even the best of intentions until more is known than we now do and until there is more political support for effective regulation. Thus far government has not evidenced much taste for firm action in the medical field.

Such disagreements obviously present difficult issues of social strategy and political judgment. Some of the advocates have recognized part of the problem in proposing, as has Senator Kennedy, that the national plan be effected in gradual steps, covering different age brackets every few years as we go along, but starting now.

Obviously there is concern about the cost of any national plan. The vagaries and intangibles of all the proposals, particularly their relative impact upon prices and utilization, make all estimates rather nebulous. Such estimates that have been made range from $12–40 billion at 1968 prices. While this would not be a net increase, since much of the money would represent a transfer from private to public channels, any adequate program will have a sizeable effect on the federal budget.

Conclusion

1. Intelligent analysis and effective control of costs must take account of the entirety of how we finance, organize, and deliver health services, as well as the external economy.

2. It would be illusory to believe that we can, or ought to, prevent health care costs from rising. The question is whether the increases can be contained, kept in reasonable relationship to the rest of the economy, sensibly commensurate with the added value of the product, and whether we can get more for our dollars through greater productivity.

3. While the health economy will expand, a higher degree of regulation seems inescapable. As increasing portions of our gross national product and more public funds go into health care, and as it exacerbates as a public issue, the demand for controls appears inevitable. The

disciplines of the competitive market economy are, for the most part, inoperative in health services.

4. As controls are instituted we will have to find more sophisticated and informative means for evaluating expenditures and their consequences: measures of productivity; more satisfactory measures of the effectiveness of different types of delivery of care and different levels of care; effects of additional inputs of resources upon the health status of the nation; relative costs of different mixes of manpower; and similar problems.

5. Whether or not we succeed in the quest for better and fairer means of financing health care, more effective and efficient delivery of services, and equitable availability of care for the entire population, we soon must face a number of issues of another dimension. Medical science and technological capabilities are inexorably expanding in geometric progression. Recent years have seen development of cures and controls of deadly diseases, but frequently they are enormously expensive. Persons with kidney failure can now be kept alive and functioning with dialysis, but at a cost of $10,000 or more a year. At present resources are available for only a small fraction of the many thousands who otherwise die of this disease. Transplants and implantation of artificial organs are at the frontier. Each involves many thousands of dollars. Many other "miracles" are in the offing. Demands for such services are incalculable.

The resources required to meet all potential demands for newly developing technologies boggle the mind; they are virtually boundless. Will the nation be forced to set limits upon health services, despite their life saving potential? How are such limits to be established? Will choices have to be made as to who will have access to these costly procedures and who will not? In an evolving culture of equal rights to health care, how will such choices be made? Who will make them?

6. It is right that our energies are now engaged in the paramount and immediate struggle to employ more effectively and equitably the great resources we invest in health services. But we must be reminded that health services do not alone bring health. It seems safe to say, for example, that even if we attain full equality in services for the poor, their health status will remain unequal. Health services will not overcome the disadvantages of poverty itself—the consequences of inferior housing, food, recreation, and education. For other classes as well, as the level of health services rises, a point of diminishing returns from such services may be reached as compared with investment in the quality of the living environment. Thus we may have to turn our attention to another aspect of the thorny question of rational allocation

of resources. In terms of health objectives, at what point is it counter-productive to invest in marginal increments to health services in preference to other social needs? The time for frankly acknowledged choices may not be far away.

Index

Abortion, and contraception, 111
Accidents, 51–52, 100
Adolescence, 22–29
Aged, care of, 99
Aid to Dependent Children, 20
Air pollution, 135
Alcoholics Anonymous, 83
Alcoholism, 61, 79–83, 100, 101
American Dental Association, 15
American Hospital Association, 81, 183, 184, 189
American Medical Association, 81, 86, 155, 199
American Psychiatric Association, 68, 76
American Psychological Association, 132
Amphetamines, 86
Antibiotics, 69, 96, 129
Anxiety neuroses, 101
Appalachia, 145
Arthritis, 158
Association of American Medical Colleges, 115, 155
Atherosclerosis, 110–11
Autonomy, 25

Barbiturates, 85, 86, 129
Barr Committee, 187, 194
Biochemical genetics, 10
Biomedical research, 96, 101–3, 105–12, 181
Biomedicine, environmental, 137
Blue Cross, 189, 195; see also Health insurance
Brain damage, 21
Bronchitis, 58, 135

Cancer, 55–57, 97, 100, 110
Cardiovascular disease, 54–55
Care of mentally ill, innovations in, 69–70
Ceiling rates, 195
Cerebral vascular disease, 157

Chemicals, hazardous, 134
Chemotherapeutic agents, 96
Child care facilities, 19, 30
Child guidance clinics, 77
Child psychiatry, 76–77
Cigarette smoking, effect on health, 100–101
Clinics, 152
Commerce, U.S. Department of, 125
Community Health Planning Act, 142
Community Health Service, National Commission on, 142
Community mental health centers, 61
Community mental health programs, 70, 72–73
Community planning, 165
Community psychiatry, 74–75
Congenital heart disease, 54
Consumer Price Index, medical care component of, 170, 172, 174
Contraception, and abortion, 111
Contraceptives, oral, 129
Coronary artery disease, 101
Coronary heart disease, 55
Crime, 132–33
Criminal responsibility, of mentally ill, 87–88
Cytogenetics, 10

Day care programs, 19
DDT, 134
Death-rate trend changes, 41–43
Degenerative disease, 99
Delinquent behavior, 26, 99–100
Dental disease, 62–63
Dental health, 14–16
Dental hygienists, increase in, 145
Dental visits, number of, 158
Dentists:
    expenditure for, 171
    increase in, 145
    number of, 143

Dentistry, 116, 125
Destructive behavior, 26, 99–100
Deviants, social, 73
Diagnostic and treatment centers, 151
Disability, 47–48, 99, 158
Disease patterns:
    as reflected by morbidity rates, 46–48
    as reflected by mortality rates, 40–43
DMT, 86
DNA, 126
Drug abuse, 83–84, 101, 104
Drug explosion, 128–29
Drugs, 70
    heart, 129
    interaction with food additives, 130–31
    out-of-hospital, 171
    psychotropic, 84
Drug use, 26, 84–87

Early learning, need for, 17–18
Ecology:
    favorable, need for, 36–37
    human, 137–39
Economic Costs of Air Pollution, 137
Economic Opportunity Act (1964), 18
Education, and research, 154–56
Emphysema, 100
Enrichment programs, for infants, 18
Environmental biomedicine, 137
Environmental Council, 36
Environmental influences, 36–37
Environment, protection of, 133–39
Experimental research, 95–96

Family planning, 9
Federal Employees Health Benefits Program, 192, 200
Flexner Report, 114
Food additives, 130
Food and Drug Administration, 85
Food, Nutrition, and Health, White House Conference on, 14, 31
Forensic psychiatry, 87–88
Fortune, 193
Functional psychoses, 61

Genetic counselling centers, 9–10
German measles, 7, 78
Germ theory, 73
Government expenditure, for medical care, 180–82

Group clinics, 151, 153, 154
Group practice, 153
Group practice plans, prepaid, 191–92
Growth, complexity of, 26–27

Hallucinogens, 84, 85, 86, 87
Handicapping conditions, minimizing of, 8–12
Headstart (see Project Headstart)
Health:
    assessment of, 39–64
    concept of, 6–7
    effect of poverty on, 12–16
    expenditures for (1968), 125
    knowledge of, 93–120
    and mental illness, 60–62
    and science, 95–98
    White House Conference on, 142
Health care:
    cost of, 167–202
    delivery of, 141–66, 168
    effectiveness of, 157–59
    essentials of, 159–61
    improvements of, 161–65
    national expenditure for, 168–71
Health education, 112–15, 163
Health, Education and Welfare, U.S. Department of, 148, 180
Health Examination Survey, 62, 63
Health facilities, 148–54
    types of, 151–54
Health goal, national, 142
Health insurance, 169, 174–79
    timing of national plan, 200–201
    universal, 197–201
Health Insurance Association of America, 189
Health maintenance, 8
Health manpower, 143–48
    National Advisory Commission on, 113, 142, 145, 191
    shortage of, 118–20
Health personnel, utilization of, 147–48
Health planning, 161–65
Health problems, 98–101
Health protection:
    nature of, 128–37
    as profession, 123–24
    resources for, 122–28
    youth involvement in, 138–39
Health protector, consumer as, 124–25
Health resources, 143

Health Resources Statistics, 112
Health services:
 distribution of, 162–63
 personal, 96, 104–5
Health worker, as nonprofessional, 124
Heart disease, 54–55, 97, 111, 158
Heart drugs, 129
Hepatitis, 135
Heterosexual relationships, 26
Highway fatalities, and alcohol, 80
Hill-Burton program, 149, 188
Homicide, 158
Hospital administration, professionalization of, 193
Hospital and Health Affairs, National Forum on, 142
Hospital Effectiveness, Advisory Committee on, 142
Hospital payments, 194–96
Hospitals:
 admission rate of, 59–60
 expenditure for, 171
 as substitute for primary physician, 150–51
Human development, concept of, 6–7
Hygiene, 99
Hypertension, 101
Hypertensive heart disease, 55

Idiosyncratic behavior, 66
Illness:
 acute, 46–47
 chronic, 47
Immunology, 110
Indolence, 100–101
Infantile paralysis, 103
Infant mortality rates, 11–12, 43–46, 98
Infection, problems of, 109–10
Influenza, 50–51, 57, 135
Injuries, from accidents, 52–53
Insomnia, 129
Institutional care, of mentally ill, 68–69
Internships, medical, 115, 118
Involuntary commitment, 66, 88
Iron-deficiency anemia, 13
Irresistible impulse, 88

Job Corps, 27

Kaiser Foundation Medical Care Program, 191, 192

Laboratory personnel, increase in, 145
Learning, early need for, 17–18
Leukemia, 56
Longevity, 33
LSD, 84, 85, 86, 87

Malnutrition, 13–14, 31
Manpower:
 development, 27
 in health field, 143–48
Marijuana, 84, 85
Measles, 49; *see also* German measles
Medicaid, 34, 129, 141, 151, 169, 177, 181, 195, 196, 199
Medical care:
 component of Consumer Price Index, 170, 172, 174
 sources of rising cost in, 182–86
 system of, 59–60
Medical centers, 116
Medical Costs, National Conference on, 142
Medical doctors (*see* Physicians)
Medical education:
 background of, 113–14
 present state of, 115
 system of, 116–17
Medical indigence, 177
Medical laboratory technologists, number of, 143
Medical research, 95–97, 125–28
 expenditure for, 96, 171
Medical specialization, 144, 160
Medicare, 34, 129, 141, 151, 169, 174, 178, 181, 189, 194, 195, 196, 198
Memorial-type hospitals, 151
Meningitis, 135
Menopause, 32
Mens rea, doctrine of, 88
Mental deficiency, 61
Mental health, 65–91
 community-oriented programs, 70, 72–73
 defined, 90
 effect of poverty on, 12–16
 nature and nurture of, 73–76
Mental Health Act (1963), 79
Mental Health of Children, Joint Commission on, 16
Mental hygiene, defined, 90
Mental Hygiene, National Committee for, 77

Mental illness:
and health, 60–62
extent of, 67–73
historical concept of, 66–67
Mentally ill, criminal responsibility of, 87–88
Mental retardation, 77–79
Metabolic diseases, 104
M'Naghten case, 87–88
Morbidity, 40–41
Morbidity rates, 157–58
disease patterns as reflected by, 46–48
Mortality, 39–40
Mortality rate, 157–58
disease patterns as reflected by, 40–43
infant, 43–46
nonwhite, 157

National Center for Health Services Research and Development, 142, 165
National Center for Health Statistics, 62, 142
National health goal, 142
National Health Insurance, Committee for, 198
National Health Survey, 15, 40, 46, 53, 58
National Institute of Health, 96, 151, 154, 165
National Institutes of Mental Health, 20, 68, 90
National insurance plan, timing of, 200–201
National Mental Health Act (1946), 69
Neighborhood health centers, 151, 154
Neoplastic disease, 110
Neuroses, anxiety, 101
Nurses:
increase in, 145
number of, 113, 143
Nursing education, 116
Nursing home care, expenditure for, 171

Obesity, 31, 100
Office of Economic Opportunity (OEO), 18, 181
Opiates, 84, 85
Opinion Research Corporation, 84
Oral contraceptives, 129

Osteopaths, number of, 113
Out-patient departments, 150
Overpopulation, and health, 98–99
Overutilization, 163–64

Parasitic infections, 109
Partnership for Health, legislation, 188
Peptic ulcer, 101
Personal health services, 96, 104–5
Personality:
development, 16
disorders, 61
Pesticides, 134
Pharmacists, number of, 143
Physical health (*see* Health)
Physician:
assistants, 147–48
hospital as substitute for, 150–51
partnerships, 151, 152
payments, 196
types of practice, 151–54
visits, 59, 158
Physicians:
expenditure for, 171
number of, 113, 143
ratio of to population, 118
shortage, 118
Planning, of medical services, 187–88
Pneumonia, 57
Poliomyelitis, 49–50, 135
Pollution:
air, 135
water, 134
Population:
explosion, 111
genetics, 10
Postdoctoral medical education, 115
Postpubescence, disorders, 24
Poverty:
effect of on physical and mental health, 12–16
and health, 98
Prenatal care, 10–11
Prepaid group practice plans, 191–92
Preprofessional medical education, 115
Prepubescence, 23–24
Preventive care, 191
Preventive detention, 66, 88
Priorities, 112
federal, 96–98
Privacy, right of, 132

Professional medical education, 115
Professional productivity, 145–47
Project Headstart, 15, 18–19
Proprietary health organizations, 190–91
Psychiatric services, 75–76
Psychological development, 24–25, 35
Psychoneuroses, 61
Psychopathology, 73, 83
Psychoses, functional, 61
Psychotropic drugs, 84
Pubescence, 23
Public Health Service, U.S., 142, 188
Pulmonary disease, 57–58, 157
Pulmonary emphysema, 100

Radiation hazard, 127, 135, 136
Rebelliousness, 26
Remedial programs, for youth, 27–28
Research:
  applied biomedical, 106–7
  basic biomedical, 105–6
  biomedical, 101–3
  and education, 154–56
  experimental, 95–96
  medical, 95–97, 125–28
Residency, medical, 115
Retirement age, 33
Rheumatic heart disease, 55
Rheumatism, 158
RNA, 126

Schizophrenia, 69
School-age child, 20
School drop-outs, 27
Science, and health, 95–98
Sedatives, 84, 85, 129
Separating experiences, 35–36
Sex education, need for, 23
Sexual psychopath, 88

Sleep, and sedatives, 129
Smoking, 100–101
Social Security Bulletin, 176
Sodium pentobarbital, 129
Solo practice, 152, 154
Somatism, 67
Stimulants, 84, 85
Stress:
  diseases of, 101
  protection against, 131–32
Strokes, 101, 111
Suicides, 102, 104
  student, 132
Survival, 93–94
Syphilis, 61
Systemization, of medical care, 186–87

Tax credit insurance plans, 199
Thalidomide, 7
Third-party payments, 196
Tobacco, and disease, 100–101
Tracheal bronchitis, 135
Tranquilizers, 70, 71, 84, 85, 129, 131
Tuberculosis, 157

Universal health insurance, 197–201
Unwed mothers, 28

Viral disease, 110

Waste disposal, 133
Water fluoridation, 15
Water pollution, 134
World Health Organization, 6, 39

X-ray technologists, increase in, 145

Youth involvement, in health protection, 138–39

The American Assembly

COLUMBIA UNIVERSITY

Trustees

Arthur G. Altschul	New York
Robert O. Anderson	New Mexico
George W. Ball	New York
William Benton	Connecticut
Courtney C. Brown, *Chairman*	New York
William P. Bundy	Massachusetts
Josephine Young Case	New York
Andrew W. Cordier, *ex officio*	New York
John Cowles	Minnesota
George S. Craft	Georgia
Marriner S. Eccles	Utah
Milton S. Eisenhower	Maryland
Arthur S. Flemming	Minnesota
Katharine Graham	District of Columbia
W. Averell Harriman	New York
Hubert H. Humphrey	Minnesota
George F. James, *ex officio*	New York
J. Erik Jonsson	Texas
Sol M. Linowitz	New York
Don G. Mitchell	New Jersey
Clifford C. Nelson, *ex officio*	New Jersey

Officers

Clifford C. Nelson, *President*
Kurt Ludwig, *Secretary*
Marian Wezmar, *Treasurer*
Mary M. McLeod, *Assistant to the President*

Chairman Emeritus

Henry M. Wriston	New York

About the American Assembly

The American Assembly was established by Dwight D. Eisenhower at Columbia University in 1950. It holds nonpartisan meetings and publishes authoritative books to illuminate issues of United States policy.

An affiliate of Columbia, with offices in the Graduate School of Business, the Assembly is a national educational institution incorporated in the State of New York.

The Assembly seeks to provide information, stimulate discussion, and evoke independent conclusions in matters of vital public interest.

AMERICAN ASSEMBLY SESSIONS

At least two national programs are initiated each year. Authorities are retained to write background papers presenting essential data and defining the main issues in each subject.

About sixty men and women representing a broad range of experience, competence, and American leadership meet for several days to discuss the Assembly topic and consider alternatives for national policy.

All Assemblies follow the same procedure. The background papers are sent to participants in advance of the Assembly. The Assembly meets in small groups for four or five lengthy periods. All groups use the same agenda. At the close of these informal sessions, participants adopt in plenary session a final report of findings and recommendations.

Regional, state, and local Assemblies are held following the national session at Arden House. Assemblies have also been held in England, Switzerland, Malaysia, Canada, the Caribbean, South America, Central America, the Philippines, and Japan. Over one hundred institutions have co-sponsored one or more Assemblies.

ARDEN HOUSE

Home of The American Assembly and scene of the national sessions is Arden House, which was given to Columbia University in 1950 by W. Averell Harriman. E. Roland Harriman joined his brother in contributing toward adaptation of the property for conference purposes. The buildings surrounding the land, known as the Harriman Campus of Columbia University, are fifty miles north of New York City.

Arden House is a distinguished conference center. It is self-supporting and operates throughout the year for use by organizations with educational objectives.

AMERICAN ASSEMBLY BOOKS

The background papers for each Assembly program are published in cloth and paperbound editions for use by individuals, libraries, businesses, public agencies, nongovernmental organizations, educational institutions, discussion and service groups. In this way the deliberations of Assembly sessions are continued and extended.

The subjects of Assembly programs to date are:

1951——United States–Western Europe Relationships
1952——Inflation
1953——Economic Security for Americans
1954——The United States' Stake in the United Nations
——The Federal Government Service
1955——United States Agriculture
——The Forty-Eight States
1956——The Representation of the United States Abroad
——The United States and the Far East
1957——International Stability and Progress
——Atoms for Power
1958——The United States and Africa
——United States Monetary Policy
1959——Wages, Prices, Profits, and Productivity
——The United States and Latin America
1960——The Federal Government and Higher Education
——The Secretary of State
——Goals for Americans
1961——Arms Control: Issues for the Public
——Outer Space: Prospects for Man and Society
1962——Automation and Technological Change
——Cultural Affairs and Foreign Relations
1963——The Population Dilemma
——The United States and the Middle East
1964——The United States and Canada
——The Congress and America's Future
1965——The Courts, the Public, and the Law Explosion
——The United States and Japan
1966——State Legislatures in American Politics
——A World of Nuclear Powers?
——The United States and the Philippines
——Challenges to Collective Bargaining
1967——The United States and Eastern Europe
——Ombudsmen for American Government?
1968——Uses of the Seas
——Law in a Changing America
——Overcoming World Hunger

1969——Black Economic Development
    ——The States and the Urban Crisis
1970——The Health of Americans
    ——The United States and the Caribbean

Second Editions, Revised:

1962——The United States and the Far East
1963——The United States and Latin America
    ——The United States and Africa
1964——United States Monetary Policy
1965——The Federal Government Service
    ——The Representation of the United States Abroad
1968——Cultural Affairs and Foreign Relations
    ——Outer Space: Prospects for Man and Society
1969——The Population Dilemma